Midnight Wellness

Sarah Chen

Published by Fiel LLC, 2024.

MIDNIGHT WELLNESS

First edition. November 14, 2024.

Copyright © 2024 Sarah Chen.

ISBN: 979-8230016878

Written by Sarah Chen.

The Night Shift Revolution: Why This Book Exists

Every night, as the world winds down and lights dim across neighborhoods, a different kind of day begins. While millions drift off to sleep, an army of essential workers springs into action, keeping our hospitals running, our streets safe, our supply chains moving, and our 24/7 world functioning. If you're reading this book, you're likely one of these nocturnal warriors, or perhaps you're preparing to join their ranks. Either way, you're part of a growing segment of society that faces unique challenges and opportunities in maintaining health, happiness, and balance while living life on an unconventional schedule.

I wrote this book because, for too long, night shift workers have been handed generic wellness advice that simply doesn't work for their reality. As a former night shift nurse who spent seven years working in emergency departments across the country, I intimately understand the frustration of being told to "just get eight hours of sleep" or "eat dinner with your family" when neither of those things align with your actual life. The existing literature on health and wellness almost exclusively caters to those working traditional hours, leaving night shift workers to cobble together their own solutions through trial and error.

The statistics tell us that approximately 20 million Americans work regular night shifts, with millions more working rotating or irregular schedules. These numbers are growing as our society becomes increasingly dependent on round the clock services. Yet despite representing such a significant portion of the workforce, night shift workers have largely been left to figure things out on their own. The consequences of this oversight are serious: studies show that night shift workers face higher risks of cardiovascular disease, digestive problems, mental health challenges, and metabolic disorders compared to their daytime counterparts.

But here's what those concerning statistics don't tell you: with the right strategies and support, it's entirely possible to thrive on the night shift. I've seen it firsthand, both in my own journey and in the hundreds of night shift workers I've coached over the past decade. The key lies in understanding that working nights isn't just about doing the same things at different times; it requires a complete reimagining of how we approach health, wellness, and life balance.

Throughout this book, we'll explore evidence based strategies specifically designed for night shift workers. You won't find any one size fits all solutions here. Instead, you'll discover flexible frameworks that can be adapted to your unique situation, whether you're a nurse working three 12 hour shifts, a security guard pulling five 8 hour nights, or anyone in between. We'll delve into the science behind circadian rhythms and learn how to work with your body's natural processes rather than against them. You'll learn how to optimize your nutrition, exercise, sleep, and social life while maintaining your mental health and family connections.

This isn't just another health book; it's a comprehensive guide to rebuilding your life around your schedule. We'll tackle practical challenges like finding healthy food options at 3 AM, creating a sleep sanctuary in broad daylight, and maintaining relationships with friends and family who live on opposite schedules. You'll hear real stories from night shift veterans who have successfully navigated these challenges, and you'll get concrete, actionable advice for implementing positive changes in your own life.

One of the most powerful aspects of night shift work that often goes unrecognized is the unique opportunity it presents for personal growth and development. The quiet hours of the night can provide unparalleled focus time for pursuing education, creative projects, or side hustles. The premium pay often associated with night work can accelerate financial goals. The camaraderie among night shift workers often creates lasting friendships and professional networks. Throughout this book, we'll explore how to maximize these advantages while minimizing the potential drawbacks of working against society's normal rhythm.

What sets this book apart is its foundation in both scientific research and real world experience. Every recommendation has been tested not just in controlled studies, but in the trenches of actual night shift work. The strategies you'll learn have been refined through feedback from thousands of night workers across various industries, from healthcare and emergency services to manufacturing and transportation. This isn't theory; it's practical wisdom that works in the real world.

As we begin this journey together, I want you to know that thriving on the night shift is not just possible; it's achievable with the right knowledge and tools. Whether you're new to night work or a seasoned veteran looking to optimize your lifestyle, this book will serve as your comprehensive guide to creating a sustainable, healthy, and fulfilling life on the night shift.

In the chapters that follow, we'll systematically address every aspect of night shift wellness, from the basics of circadian rhythm adaptation to advanced strategies for long term success. We'll explore how to handle holidays, vacations, and special occasions without compromising your health or missing out on important moments. You'll learn how to create emergency protocols for unexpected schedule changes and how to navigate the unique challenges of rotating shifts.

Remember, choosing to work nights whether by necessity or preference doesn't mean you have to sacrifice your health, happiness, or quality of life. With the right approach, you can build a lifestyle that not only works but allows you to thrive. Welcome to your guide to midnight wellness; let's begin the journey to transforming your night shift experience from surviving to thriving.

Understanding Your New Normal: The Science of Working Against Nature

W orking against our natural circadian rhythm isn't just a matter of staying awake when others sleep; it represents a fundamental challenge to our biology that requires understanding and strategic adaptation. As humans, we evolved over millions of years to be active during daylight hours and rest during darkness. This chapter explores the scientific foundations of why working nights feels so challenging and what happens in your body when you attempt to reverse its natural patterns.

At the most basic level, humans are diurnal creatures, meaning we're biologically programmed to be active during the day and sleep at night. This programming runs deep, affecting everything from our hormone production to our digestion, body temperature, and cognitive function. When you work nights, you're essentially asking your body to function in direct opposition to millions of years of evolutionary programming.

The human body operates on numerous biological rhythms, with the circadian rhythm being the most prominent. This internal clock is regulated by a small region in your brain called the suprachiasmatic nucleus (SCN), which responds primarily to light and darkness. When your eyes detect light, particularly blue wavelengths, the SCN signals your body to suppress melatonin production and increase cortisol, preparing you for wakefulness and activity. Darkness triggers the opposite response, promoting melatonin production and preparing your body for rest.

This biological programming creates what scientists call "process C" the circadian rhythm and "process S" the sleep pressure that builds the longer you're awake. Under normal circumstances, these two processes work in harmony, making you feel alert during daylight hours and sleepy at night. When you work nights, you're forcing these processes out of alignment, creating what researchers call circadian misalignment.

The consequences of this misalignment manifest in various ways. Your body temperature, which naturally drops during nighttime hours to facilitate sleep, must now remain elevated when you're working. Your digestive system, which typically slows during the night, must process meals when it's programmed for rest. Even your liver, which plays a crucial role in metabolism and detoxification, operates on its own circadian rhythm that becomes disrupted.

Understanding these biological challenges is crucial because it helps explain why simply trying to "power through" night shifts often leads to burnout and health problems. Your body isn't fighting against you out of stubbornness; it's responding to deeply ingrained biological programming that has ensured human survival for generations.

The good news is that while we can't completely override our natural biology, we can work with it to create sustainable adaptations. Research has shown that the human body possesses remarkable plasticity in its circadian rhythms. While complete reversal of our natural patterns may not be possible, we can achieve a workable compromise through strategic light exposure, carefully timed meals, and consistent sleep schedules.

One of the most significant challenges night workers face is light exposure. Our bodies interpret light, particularly sunlight, as a powerful wake signal. When you leave work in the morning, your body receives an intense blast of sunlight just when you need to be winding down for sleep. This creates what scientists call circadian confusion, where your internal clock receives conflicting signals about whether it should be promoting wakefulness or rest.

Temperature regulation presents another biological challenge. Your body temperature naturally drops during the night hours, reaching its lowest point typically between 2 AM and 4 AM. When working nights, you need to maintain alertness during this natural trough. Understanding this helps explain why night workers often feel coldest during these hours and why it's particularly challenging to stay alert during this time.

Hormone production follows its own circadian pattern, with cortisol (the stress hormone that promotes wakefulness) typically peaking in the early morning hours and declining throughout the day. Melatonin, the sleep hormone, typically begins rising in the evening and peaks in the middle of the night. When working nights, you're essentially asking these hormones to reverse their natural patterns, which takes time and consistent behavior to achieve even partial adaptation.

Digestion and metabolism also operate on circadian rhythms. Your insulin sensitivity is naturally lower at night, meaning your body processes carbohydrates differently during these hours. Your stomach produces less acid, and your intestinal motility slows. This explains why many night workers experience digestive issues and why eating the wrong foods at the wrong times can lead to significant discomfort.

Understanding these biological challenges helps explain why traditional health advice often fails night shift workers. When someone suggests "just getting eight hours of sleep," they're not accounting for the complex biological processes that make daytime sleep fundamentally different from nighttime sleep. When they recommend "eating dinner at normal times," they're not considering how this conflicts with your body's metabolic rhythms.

The key to success lies in working with your biology rather than against it. Throughout this book, we'll explore specific strategies for managing these biological challenges, but the foundation begins with understanding. When you know why your body responds the way it does, you can make informed decisions about how to adjust your lifestyle to support your health while working nights.

Remember that while our biology presents challenges to night work, humans have demonstrated remarkable adaptability throughout history. The key is not to fight against your natural rhythms but to work with them, creating new patterns that support your health while meeting the demands of your schedule. In the chapters that follow, we'll build on this foundation of understanding to develop practical strategies for managing every aspect of night shift life.

Think of this adaptation process as learning to dance with your biology rather than wrestling against it. You may not be able to completely change the music your body wants to play, but you can learn new steps that allow you to move gracefully within the constraints of night work while maintaining your health and wellbeing.

Circadian Rhythms: Your Internal Clock Explained

Your circadian rhythm is more than just a biological clock; it's an intricate system of molecular processes that governs nearly every aspect of your physiology. Understanding how this internal timekeeper works is crucial for anyone attempting to adapt to night shift work. Let's dive deep into the mechanics of your circadian rhythm and explore how it influences your daily functioning.

At its core, your circadian rhythm operates through a complex network of genes and proteins that create a roughly 24-hour cycle of biological processes. This cycle isn't just about sleep and wakefulness; it regulates hormone production, body temperature, metabolism, immune function, and even cognitive performance. The primary conductor of this biological orchestra is a small cluster of neurons in your brain's hypothalamus called the suprachiasmatic nucleus (SCN).

The SCN receives direct input from your eyes through a specialized pathway that's separate from your visual system. This pathway is particularly sensitive to blue light wavelengths, which is why exposure to sunlight or electronic devices can have such a powerful effect on your alertness levels. When light hits specialized cells in your retina, they send signals to the SCN, which then coordinates various biological processes throughout your body.

One of the most important outputs of your circadian system is the regulation of melatonin, often called the sleep hormone. Under normal circumstances, melatonin production begins to increase in the evening hours, peaks in the middle of the night, and decreases toward morning. This pattern helps explain why you naturally feel sleepy at night and alert during the day. However, melatonin isn't just about sleep; it also plays crucial roles in immune function, antioxidant protection, and metabolic regulation.

Your circadian rhythm also controls the production of cortisol, the stress hormone that helps you wake up and maintain alertness. Cortisol typically peaks in the early morning hours, helping you naturally wake up and prepare for the day ahead. This hormone follows a predictable pattern called the cortisol awakening response (CAR), which can become disrupted when working nights.

Temperature regulation is another crucial function of your circadian rhythm. Your core body temperature fluctuates throughout the day, typically reaching its peak in the late afternoon and its lowest point in the early morning hours. This temperature rhythm has important implications for sleep quality and cognitive performance. When you try to sleep during the day, you're often fighting against your body's natural temperature peak, which can make it harder to fall asleep and stay asleep.

Your metabolic processes also follow circadian patterns. Insulin sensitivity, glucose tolerance, and lipid metabolism all vary throughout the day. This is why eating at unusual times can affect how your body processes nutrients. Your digestive system produces different levels of enzymes and acids at different times of the day, which can impact how well you digest and absorb nutrients from your food.

The circadian system operates through what scientists call "clock genes," which are present in virtually every cell of your body. These genes create feedback loops that turn various biological processes on and off throughout the day. This means that different organs and systems in your body have their own internal clocks, all of which are normally synchronized by the master clock in your SCN.

When you work night shifts, you're essentially asking all these individual clocks to reset themselves to a new schedule. This process, known as entrainment, doesn't happen instantaneously. Different systems in your body adapt at different rates, which can lead to what researchers call internal desynchronization. This desynchronization helps explain many of the symptoms night shift workers experience, from digestive issues to mood disturbances.

Your circadian rhythm isn't just influenced by light; it responds to other environmental cues called zeitgebers. These include meal timing, physical activity, social interactions, and temperature changes. Understanding these various influences gives you multiple tools for helping your body adjust to a night shift schedule. By carefully timing your exposure to different zeitgebers, you can help your circadian system adapt more effectively to your work schedule.

It's important to note that circadian rhythms have a genetic component. Some people are naturally "night owls" while others are "morning larks." This genetic variation can influence how well you adapt to night shift work. However, regardless of your natural chronotype, your circadian system maintains some degree of flexibility that allows for adaptation to different schedules.

The relationship between your circadian rhythm and sleep is complex. While your circadian system promotes sleepiness at certain times, it also maintains periods of heightened alertness, even when you're sleep deprived. These alertness windows can be particularly important for night shift workers to identify and utilize effectively.

Understanding your circadian rhythm also helps explain why consistent schedules are so important for night shift workers. Your body's internal clock prefers regularity and can maintain a shifted schedule more easily than it can handle frequent changes. This is why rotating shifts or irregular schedules can be particularly challenging for your health and wellbeing.

Your circadian system also influences cognitive function, including attention, memory, and decision-making abilities. This explains why you might feel mentally foggy during certain hours of your night shift, particularly during the circadian low point in the early morning hours. Understanding these patterns can help you plan your work activities more effectively, scheduling complex tasks for times when your cognitive function is naturally higher.

As we continue through this book, we'll build upon this understanding of circadian rhythms to develop practical strategies for managing night shift work. Remember that while you can't completely override your circadian rhythm, you can work with it to create a sustainable pattern that supports your health and performance during night shifts.

The First Two Weeks: Surviving the Initial Transition

The first two weeks of transitioning to night shift work represent one of the most challenging periods in a shift worker's career. During this time, your body and mind are actively fighting against years of ingrained patterns, and success depends largely on your ability to stay committed to the transition process while managing the inevitable difficulties that arise.

The initial shock to your system typically begins with your first overnight shift. Even if you've prepared by adjusting your sleep schedule gradually in the days leading up to the transition, your body will likely protest against staying awake all night. You may experience waves of intense fatigue, particularly during the circadian low point between 2 AM and 6 AM. This is completely normal and expected. During these first few nights, your primary goal should be maintaining wakefulness and safety rather than peak performance.

Physical symptoms during the first week often include digestive issues, headaches, and a general feeling of malaise. Your appetite signals may become confused, leading to unusual cravings or a complete lack of hunger at times when you know you should eat. Many night shift workers report feeling slightly dizzy or disconnected from reality during this initial period, almost as if they're moving through a fog. These sensations typically peak around day three or four of the transition.

Sleep quality during the first week is usually poor, even if you're following all the recommended protocols for daytime sleep. You might find yourself waking up frequently, experiencing vivid dreams, or feeling unrested despite getting adequate hours of sleep. This is your body's natural response to the circadian disruption, and while uncomfortable, it's temporary. The key is to maintain strict sleep hygiene practices even when it feels like they're not working. Consistency during this period lays the groundwork for better sleep in the weeks to come.

The second week typically brings some improvement in physical symptoms, but new challenges often emerge. This is when many night workers face their first real test of social adaptation. The reality of missing family dinners, daytime social events, and normal daily routines becomes more apparent. It's common to experience feelings of isolation or mild depression during this period, even if you're generally a positive person.

During this crucial second week, your body begins showing signs of adaptation to the new schedule. You might notice periods of natural alertness during your night shift, particularly if you've been consistent with your sleep schedule and light exposure patterns. However, this adaptation isn't linear. Many workers experience what we call the "false start" phenomenon, where they feel great for a day or two, only to crash harder the following night.

Managing energy levels during these first two weeks requires a strategic approach. Relying too heavily on caffeine can backfire, as it may interfere with your daytime sleep and create a cycle of increasing fatigue. Instead, focus on using light exposure, physical movement, and proper nutrition to maintain alertness. Short walks, stretching sessions, or light exercises during your breaks can help combat the intense drowsiness that typically hits during the pre-dawn hours.

Nutrition plays a crucial role during the transition period. Your digestive system needs time to adjust to the new eating schedule, so it's best to start with easily digestible meals and snacks. Many night workers make the mistake of loading up on sugar and simple carbohydrates during these first two weeks, seeking quick energy boosts. While this might provide temporary relief, it ultimately makes the adaptation process more difficult by creating blood sugar instability.

Family and social relationships require careful attention during this period. Clear communication about your needs and limitations is essential. Many night workers find it helpful to schedule specific times for family interaction, even if they're brief, to maintain connection during the transition. This might mean having breakfast with your spouse before you go to sleep, or setting aside time to video chat with children after they get home from school, even if it means interrupting your sleep schedule slightly.

The psychological aspects of the transition are often underestimated. The first two weeks can feel incredibly isolating, as you're awake when most of your social network is asleep. This is when having a support system of other night shift workers becomes invaluable. Whether through online communities or workplace connections, sharing experiences with others who understand your challenges can provide crucial emotional support.

It's important to remember that the first two weeks are not indicative of how you'll feel long-term on the night shift. Many workers who struggle intensely during this period go on to adapt successfully and even prefer night work once they've fully adjusted. The key is to view these two weeks as a temporary phase of adaptation rather than a permanent state.

By the end of the second week, most night shift workers begin to see some stabilization in their sleep patterns and energy levels. While complete adaptation typically takes longer, this two-week mark often represents a turning point where the most acute symptoms begin to subside. You might notice that you're able to sleep for longer periods during the day, and that your energy levels during your shift become more predictable.

Success during this critical period depends largely on your preparation and mindset. Those who approach the transition with a clear plan and realistic expectations typically fare better than those who try to wing it. This includes having your sleep environment properly set up before beginning night shifts, meal planning for at least the first week, and arranging support from family members or roommates to minimize daytime disruptions.

Remember that everyone's adaptation period is different, and comparing your experience to others' isn't helpful. Some people may adjust more quickly, while others might take longer to find their rhythm. The goal during these first two weeks isn't to feel perfect; it's to establish the foundational habits and routines that will support your long-term success on the night shift.

Mapping Your New Schedule: Creating Your 24-Hour Framework

C reating a sustainable schedule when working night shifts requires careful planning and consideration of your body's natural rhythms and your life obligations. The 24-hour framework you develop will serve as the foundation for your success in adapting to and thriving on the night shift.

The first step in mapping your schedule is understanding that you can't simply flip your existing routine upside down. Night shift workers who attempt to maintain the exact same schedule as day workers, just shifted by 12 hours, often struggle unnecessarily. Instead, you need to create a custom framework that accounts for the unique challenges of working against society's standard schedule.

Begin by identifying your non-negotiable time blocks. Your work hours are obviously fixed, but you also need to consider key family commitments, such as children's school schedules or regular medical appointments. These anchor points will help determine how to structure the rest of your day. Many successful night workers find that splitting their sleep into two segments allows them to participate in both nighttime work activities and daytime family obligations.

Your main sleep period should ideally be scheduled for the same time each day. Consistency is crucial for establishing healthy sleep patterns. Most night shift workers find their best sleep occurs between 9 AM and 4 PM, with the specific timing depending on their shift hours and personal circumstances. Consider factors like neighborhood noise levels, natural light patterns, and family schedules when selecting your primary sleep window.

The hours immediately before and after your main sleep period are critical transition times that require careful planning. Establish a pre-sleep routine that begins at least an hour before your intended bedtime. This might include activities like darkening your bedroom, light stretching, or reading. Similarly, plan a wake-up routine that helps energize you for your upcoming shift.

Meal timing becomes particularly important when working nights. Your framework should include designated times for substantial meals, typically one before your shift begins and another during your "lunch" break. Many night workers benefit from eating their largest meal of the day when they wake up, around 4 or 5 PM, followed by a moderate meal during their shift break, and a light meal before bed.

Exercise scheduling requires special consideration within your 24-hour framework. The optimal time for vigorous exercise is usually 4-6 hours before your main sleep period. This allows your body temperature and stress hormone levels to return to baseline before sleep. For many night workers, this means exercising either right after waking up or toward the end of their shift.

Social time must be intentionally built into your framework rather than left to chance. Designate specific hours for family interaction, friend meetups, and personal hobbies. Many successful night workers reserve early evening hours for family dinner before heading to work, or schedule regular weekend activities during their normal waking hours.

Your framework should also include buffer zones - flexible periods that can absorb unexpected schedule disruptions without completely derailing your routine. These might be used for occasional daytime appointments, family emergencies, or social events that don't align perfectly with your usual schedule.

Consider creating different versions of your framework for workdays versus days off. While maintaining the same sleep-wake schedule throughout the week is ideal, it's not always practical or desirable. Having a modified framework for days off allows you to participate in more daytime activities while minimizing circadian disruption.

Technology can be a valuable tool in maintaining your schedule. Use your phone's calendar to block out your framework, setting recurring reminders for sleep times, meals, and other daily activities. Many night workers find that sharing their digital calendar with family members helps reduce scheduling conflicts and misunderstandings.

Season changes should be factored into your framework, especially if you live in an area with significant variation in daylight hours. You might need slightly different schedules for summer versus winter months to account for changes in natural light exposure and temperature patterns.

Remember that your framework should be treated as a flexible guide rather than an rigid schedule. While consistency is important, being too strict can create unnecessary stress when life inevitably throws curveballs. The goal is to have a reliable structure that can bend without breaking.

Regular review and adjustment of your framework is essential. Set aside time every few months to evaluate how well your schedule is working and make necessary modifications. Pay attention to patterns in your energy levels, sleep quality, and overall wellbeing as indicators of whether your framework needs refinement.

Documentation can help you optimize your framework over time. Keep a log of how you feel during different parts of your schedule, noting particularly successful days as well as challenging ones. This information becomes invaluable when making adjustments to your routine.

Communicate your framework clearly to friends and family. Help them understand that your schedule isn't just a matter of preference but a carefully designed system that supports your health and performance. The more they understand your needs, the better they can support your success on the night shift.

Your 24-hour framework is more than just a schedule - it's a tool for creating stability in a lifestyle that often feels inherently unstable.

When designed thoughtfully and maintained consistently, it becomes the foundation upon which you can build a sustainable and satisfying night shift career.

Your Body on Night Shift: Physiological Changes and Adaptations

Working the night shift triggers profound changes in your body's physiological systems. Understanding these adaptations is crucial for managing your health and optimizing your performance during overnight hours. Your body wasn't naturally designed to be active at night, but it possesses remarkable abilities to adjust to this alternative schedule.

The most immediate and noticeable change occurs in your endocrine system, particularly in the production and timing of key hormones. Melatonin, often called the sleep hormone, typically increases in the evening and decreases in the morning in response to natural light patterns. When working nights, this pattern becomes disrupted, requiring your body to establish new production rhythms. Cortisol, your primary stress hormone, follows a similar pattern of disruption, potentially affecting everything from your energy levels to your immune function.

Your digestive system also undergoes significant adjustments when working nights. The stomach and intestines have their own circadian rhythms, affecting enzyme production, nutrient absorption, and waste elimination. Many night workers experience changes in appetite and digestion, particularly during the first few months of adjustment. Your metabolism may slow during nighttime hours when it's programmed to rest, potentially affecting how your body processes nutrients and stores fat.

Temperature regulation presents another physiological challenge. Your body temperature naturally drops during the night and rises during the day, regardless of your activity level. Night shift workers must function at peak performance when their core temperature is programmed to be at its lowest. This can affect muscle function, mental alertness, and overall energy levels. Your body gradually adapts by adjusting its temperature rhythm, but this process can take several weeks or even months.

Cardiovascular function also undergoes notable changes during night work. Blood pressure typically follows a daily rhythm, dropping during sleep and rising during waking hours. Night shift workers often experience alterations in this pattern, which can impact heart health over time. The heart must work harder to maintain proper circulation when active during its programmed rest period, potentially leading to increased cardiovascular stress.

Your immune system faces unique challenges when working nights. The production and activity of immune cells follow circadian patterns, with certain components being more active during normal sleep hours. Disrupting these patterns can temporarily reduce immune function, making night workers more susceptible to illness during the adaptation period. However, the body generally develops compensatory mechanisms over time.

The visual system experiences particular stress during night work. Your eyes must adapt to artificial lighting conditions when they're programmed for darkness, potentially leading to eye strain and fatigue. The photoreceptors in your retina play a crucial role in regulating your circadian rhythm, and exposure to artificial light during night shifts can either help or hinder your adaptation depending on the timing and intensity.

Muscle function and physical performance capabilities fluctuate throughout the 24-hour cycle. Night workers often notice changes in their strength, endurance, and coordination during overnight hours. This is partly due to variations in hormone levels, body temperature, and neural activation patterns. Understanding these fluctuations helps in planning physical activities and managing workload during your shift.

Your respiratory system also adapts to night work. Breathing patterns naturally change during the night, and working during these hours requires your respiratory system to maintain daytime levels of oxygen exchange when it would typically be in a reduced state. This adaptation is particularly important for workers in physically demanding jobs.

Cognitive function undergoes significant changes during night work. The brain's processing speed, attention span, and decision-making capabilities are naturally reduced during nighttime hours. While these functions can adapt to some degree, many night workers notice persistent differences in their mental performance compared to daytime functioning. This makes it crucial to develop strategies for maintaining alertness and mental acuity.

The reproductive system can be affected by night shift work, particularly in women. Menstrual cycles may become irregular due to hormonal disruptions, and fertility can be temporarily impacted. These effects typically normalize as the body adapts to the new schedule, but they represent important considerations for workers planning families.

Your kidney function and fluid balance also adjust to night work. The kidneys typically reduce urine production during sleep hours, but this pattern must shift when working nights. This adaptation affects how your body processes fluids and maintains electrolyte balance, influencing both hydration needs and bathroom frequency during your shift.

Understanding these physiological changes helps explain many of the challenges night workers face and informs strategies for managing them effectively. Your body possesses remarkable adaptive capabilities, but these adaptations take time and require consistent support through appropriate lifestyle choices. The key is working with your body's natural tendencies while gradually encouraging new patterns that better align with your work schedule.

The most successful night shift workers learn to recognize and respond to their body's signals during this adaptation process. They understand that certain physiological changes are normal and temporary, while others require ongoing management strategies. This knowledge allows them to make informed decisions about sleep, nutrition, exercise, and other lifestyle factors that support their body's adjustment to night work.

Remember that individual responses to night shift work vary significantly. Some people adapt more readily than others due to genetic factors, age, overall health status, and previous experience with varying schedules. Monitoring your own body's responses and adjustments helps you develop personalized strategies for maintaining optimal health while working nights.

The Night Shift Nutrition Foundation

Nutrition forms the cornerstone of health and performance for night shift workers, yet traditional dietary advice rarely accounts for the unique demands of working while others sleep. The foundations of night shift nutrition require a complete reimagining of conventional meal timing, food choices, and eating patterns to support your reversed schedule.

Your nutritional needs during night work differ significantly from those of day workers. The body processes nutrients differently during nighttime hours, with insulin sensitivity and metabolic rate following circadian patterns that can affect how you utilize the food you consume. Understanding these differences allows you to make strategic dietary choices that support your energy levels and overall health.

The first principle of night shift nutrition centers on maintaining stable blood sugar levels throughout your shift. When working nights, your body naturally resists processing carbohydrates as efficiently as it would during daylight hours. This resistance can lead to energy crashes and increased fat storage if not properly managed. Complex carbohydrates, combined with adequate protein and healthy fats, become essential for sustaining energy without triggering the dramatic blood sugar fluctuations that often plague night workers.

Protein takes on heightened importance during night shifts. Your muscles and organs need consistent protein availability to maintain function and repair during hours when your body would typically be at rest. Aim for protein-rich foods at regular intervals throughout your shift, focusing on sources that provide a complete amino acid profile. This helps maintain muscle mass and supports cognitive function during the challenging overnight hours.

Healthy fats play a crucial role in night shift nutrition by providing sustained energy and supporting hormone production. Your endocrine system faces unique challenges during night work, and dietary fats provide the building blocks needed for hormone synthesis. Choose sources rich in omega-3 fatty acids and monounsaturated fats while limiting saturated and trans fats that can contribute to inflammation and metabolic disruption.

Micronutrient intake requires special attention when working nights. Vitamin D deficiency becomes a particular concern since night workers often have limited sun exposure. While supplementation may be necessary, focusing on food sources rich in vitamin D, along with other essential vitamins and minerals, helps support immune function and overall health. Dark leafy greens, colorful vegetables, and nutrient-dense fruits become invaluable additions to your dietary foundation.

Fiber intake often suffers among night shift workers due to limited food options and disrupted eating patterns. Yet adequate fiber becomes even more crucial when working nights, as it helps regulate digestion and maintains gut health despite the schedule-induced challenges to your digestive system. Incorporating whole grains, legumes, and high-fiber vegetables helps prevent the constipation and digestive issues common among night workers.

The timing of your meals plays a crucial role in establishing effective night shift nutrition. Your largest meal should typically come before your shift begins, providing the energy needed for the work ahead while allowing adequate time for digestion. Smaller, nutrient-dense meals or snacks throughout your shift help maintain energy levels without overwhelming your digestive system during hours when it naturally wants to slow down.

Anti-inflammatory foods take on special significance in night shift nutrition. The disruption to your natural circadian rhythm can increase systemic inflammation, potentially contributing to various health issues over time. Foods rich in antioxidants and natural anti-inflammatory compounds help combat this effect. Berries, leafy greens, fatty fish, and nuts become powerful allies in maintaining long-term health.

Meal preparation becomes a critical skill for successful night shift nutrition. The limited availability of healthy food options during overnight hours means planning ahead becomes essential. Learning to prepare and properly store nutrient-dense meals that can be easily transported and consumed during your shift helps maintain dietary quality despite the challenges of your schedule.

Understanding the role of hunger signals during night work helps establish healthy eating patterns. Your natural hunger cues may become disrupted when working nights, making it important to develop a structured approach to eating that doesn't rely solely on appetite. Regular meal timing, based on your work schedule rather than traditional mealtimes, helps maintain consistent energy levels and supports metabolic health.

The quality of your food choices becomes increasingly important during night work. Processed foods, while convenient, often contribute to inflammation and energy crashes that can make night shifts more challenging. Focus on whole, minimally processed foods that provide sustained energy and nutritional support for your body's adapted rhythms.

Building a strong nutritional foundation for night shift work requires patience and experimentation. What works well for one person may not suit another, making it important to monitor your body's responses and adjust accordingly. Pay attention to how different foods affect your energy levels, digestion, and overall wellbeing during your shifts.

Remember that nutrition represents just one component of your overall night shift wellness strategy, but it's one that profoundly affects all others. The food choices you make influence your sleep quality, exercise performance, mental clarity, and long-term health. By establishing solid nutritional foundations specific to night work, you create the energy and vitality needed to thrive on your unconventional schedule.

Strategic Meal Timing for Overnight Workers

Strategic meal timing represents one of the most crucial yet challenging aspects of maintaining health while working overnight hours. The conventional wisdom around when to eat breaks down entirely when your active hours occur while most of the world sleeps, requiring a complete reimagining of meal scheduling to support your reversed lifestyle.

The first step in developing an effective meal timing strategy involves understanding your new metabolic patterns. Your body's ability to process and utilize nutrients fluctuates throughout the 24-hour cycle, with insulin sensitivity and digestive efficiency typically lower during nighttime hours. This natural variation means that simply shifting traditional meal times by twelve hours won't provide optimal results.

Begin by establishing your "metabolic morning" approximately one to two hours before your shift starts. This represents your body's equivalent of breakfast, though it may occur in the afternoon or evening by conventional standards. This meal should be substantial but not heavy, providing the energy needed for your upcoming shift while allowing adequate time for digestion before the demanding hours ahead.

During your actual shift, smaller, more frequent meals often prove more effective than traditional large meals. This approach helps maintain steady energy levels while preventing the digestive discomfort that can occur when consuming large amounts of food during hours when your digestive system naturally wants to slow down. Aim to eat every three to four hours during your shift, with portion sizes that satisfy hunger without causing sluggishness.

The timing of your last shift meal requires careful consideration. Eating too close to your bedtime can interfere with sleep quality, yet going to bed hungry often leads to disrupted rest. As a general rule, try to consume your final meal at least two to three hours before you plan to sleep. This meal should be lighter than your pre-shift meal but substantial enough to prevent hunger from waking you during your rest period.

Protein timing becomes especially important when working nights. Your muscles need regular protein availability for maintenance and repair, but large amounts of protein too close to bedtime can interfere with sleep. Consider concentrating your protein intake during the early and middle portions of your shift, tapering off as you approach your sleep window.

Carbohydrate timing also plays a crucial role in energy management during night shifts. Complex carbohydrates work well in your pre-shift meal and during the first half of your shift, providing sustained energy when you need it most. As your shift progresses, gradually reduce carbohydrate intake and shift toward proteins and healthy fats to maintain stable blood sugar levels without interfering with upcoming sleep.

Strategic snacking between main meals helps bridge energy gaps during long night shifts. The key lies in choosing nutrient-dense options that provide sustained energy without causing blood sugar spikes. Time these snacks to coincide with periods when you typically experience energy dips, often around the midpoint of your shift or during the challenging hours between 2 and 4 AM.

Hydration timing deserves special attention in your meal planning strategy. While staying hydrated remains crucial, timing your fluid intake can help prevent sleep disruption from bathroom visits during your rest period. Consider frontloading your hydration during the early parts of your shift, gradually tapering off as you approach your sleep window while still maintaining adequate fluid intake.

For those who exercise while working nights, meal timing becomes even more critical. If you work out before your shift, ensure you consume adequate carbohydrates and protein within an hour after completing your exercise session. For post-shift workouts, consider a small pre-exercise snack and plan your main recovery meal as part of your wind-down routine.

Adapting your meal timing for days off presents another challenge. While maintaining your night shift eating schedule during off days helps preserve your body's adapted rhythms, social obligations and family life often make this impractical. Develop a flexible transition strategy that allows you to adjust your meal timing without completely disrupting your metabolic patterns.

The role of fasting windows within your night shift schedule warrants consideration. Some workers find success with time-restricted feeding patterns that align with their work hours, while others need more frequent fueling to maintain energy and focus. Experiment with different feeding windows while monitoring your energy levels and performance to find what works best for your body.

Remember that seasonal changes can affect optimal meal timing strategies. Longer or shorter daylight hours might influence when you sleep and consequently when you eat. Remain flexible in adjusting your meal schedule to accommodate these natural variations while maintaining the core principles of night shift nutrition.

Success with strategic meal timing requires planning and preparation. Develop systems for food preparation and storage that ensure you have appropriate meals and snacks available when needed during your shift. This might mean investing in quality food storage containers and learning to prepare meals that taste good even after reheating at unusual hours.

Above all, recognize that finding your optimal meal timing strategy requires patience and experimentation. Pay attention to how different timing patterns affect your energy levels, digestion, sleep quality, and overall wellbeing. Keep a food and energy journal during this process to identify patterns and make informed adjustments to your scheduling strategy.

The 3 AM Food Guide: What to Eat and Avoid

The dreaded 3 AM hunger pangs represent one of the most challenging aspects of working overnight hours. While most of the world sleeps peacefully, night shift workers face difficult decisions about what to eat during these crucial hours when both metabolism and judgment can be compromised. Understanding how to navigate these challenging hours with proper nutrition can make the difference between thriving on your shift and struggling through it.

During the early morning hours, particularly between 2 and 4 AM, your body experiences its lowest point in terms of core temperature and energy levels. This natural dip in your circadian rhythm can trigger cravings for sugary, high carbohydrate foods that promise quick energy but ultimately lead to crashes and disrupted sleep patterns. The key lies in choosing foods that provide steady, sustainable energy while supporting your body's natural processes.

Protein becomes your greatest ally during these challenging hours. Lean protein sources like Greek yogurt, hard boiled eggs, or turkey help maintain stable blood sugar levels while providing the amino acids your body needs for repair and maintenance. These proteins also contain tryptophan, which can help regulate your sleep wake cycle when you finally head to bed after your shift.

Complex carbohydrates play a supporting role during the 3 AM period, but selection and portion size prove crucial. While your body might crave simple sugars, choosing whole grain options like oatmeal, quinoa, or brown rice provides steady energy without the spike and crash associated with processed carbohydrates. Combine these complex carbohydrates with protein and healthy fats to create balanced mini meals that sustain you through the remainder of your shift.

Healthy fats deserve special attention during these hours. Foods rich in omega-3 fatty acids and medium chain triglycerides provide sustained energy while supporting cognitive function when your body naturally wants to slow down. Nuts, seeds, avocados, and olive oil make excellent additions to your early morning fuel strategy. These fats help you feel satisfied without the heaviness that can come from larger meals.

Certain foods should be strictly avoided during the 3 AM period. Processed snacks, sugary beverages, and heavy, greasy foods can wreak havoc on your digestion and energy levels. These foods are particularly problematic during night hours when your digestive system naturally slows down. The temporary satisfaction they provide quickly gives way to discomfort and lethargy that can make the remainder of your shift particularly challenging.

Portion control becomes especially important during these hours. Your body's ability to process and utilize nutrients efficiently decreases during the night, making smaller, more frequent meals preferable to large portions. Aim for snack sized portions that provide around 200-300 calories, combining multiple food groups to ensure balanced nutrition without overwhelming your digestive system.

Preparation proves essential for successful 3 AM nutrition. Having healthy options readily available prevents the temptation to visit vending machines or grab processed snacks from convenience stores. Pack portable, nutrient dense foods that require minimal preparation and can be easily consumed during brief breaks. Consider investing in quality food storage containers that keep foods at proper temperatures throughout your shift.

Hydration choices during these hours significantly impact your energy levels and subsequent sleep quality. While caffeine might seem like an obvious choice, its consumption during the early morning hours can interfere with your ability to rest after your shift. Instead, focus on water, herbal teas, and electrolyte beverages that support hydration without disrupting your sleep patterns. If you must consume caffeine, limit it to the earlier portions of your shift.

Temperature and texture of foods can influence their effectiveness during these challenging hours. Many night workers find that room temperature or slightly cool foods prove easier to digest than very hot or cold options. Incorporating a variety of textures can help maintain interest in healthy choices when fatigue might otherwise lead to poor food decisions. Consider combining crunchy vegetables with creamy dips or adding nuts to yogurt for textural contrast.

Social eating during these hours presents another challenge. When colleagues order takeout or bring in shared snacks, maintaining healthy choices becomes more difficult. Develop strategies for navigating these situations while staying true to your nutrition goals. This might mean keeping portion controlled alternatives readily available or learning to politely decline while explaining your commitment to supporting your health through proper nutrition.

The psychological aspects of eating during these hours cannot be ignored. Many workers struggle with emotional eating during the 3 AM period when fatigue and stress levels peak. Developing alternative coping mechanisms for stress and establishing clear boundaries around comfort eating helps maintain healthy patterns during these vulnerable hours. Consider keeping a food journal to identify emotional eating triggers and develop more constructive responses.

Emergency nutrition planning for the 3 AM period proves essential for long term success. Despite best intentions, situations will arise when your planned foods aren't available or accessible. Maintain a small stash of shelf stable, nutrient dense options in your locker or work area. These emergency options should still align with your overall nutrition goals while providing the energy needed to complete your shift effectively.

Remember that the 3 AM period represents a temporary challenge within your shift. The foods you choose during these hours impact not only your immediate performance but also your ability to rest effectively when your shift ends. By approaching this challenging time with planning, preparation, and knowledge about optimal food choices, you can maintain energy levels and support your overall health while working against your body's natural rhythms.

Meal Prep Strategies for Night Shift Success

S uccess on the night shift requires a well-planned approach to meal preparation that accounts for the unique challenges of working unconventional hours. Without proper planning and preparation, night workers often find themselves relying on unhealthy convenience foods or struggling to maintain consistent nutrition throughout their shifts.

The foundation of successful meal prep for night shift workers begins with understanding the optimal timing of meal preparation sessions. Most night shift workers find success by dedicating one or two days to bulk preparation when they are most alert and energized. This typically means preparing meals either before starting a stretch of night shifts or during recovery days. The key is identifying when you personally have the most energy and motivation to tackle meal preparation tasks.

Creating a meal prep routine requires careful consideration of food storage and reheating facilities available at your workplace. Many night shift workers have limited access to full kitchens, often relying on microwaves and small refrigerators. This reality should inform your choice of recipes and storage containers. Invest in high quality, microwave safe containers that seal properly to prevent leaks and maintain freshness. Consider containers with divided compartments to keep foods separated and maintain proper textures.

When planning your meal prep sessions, focus on recipes that hold up well over several days and can be enjoyed at room temperature if necessary. Cold grain bowls, protein packed salads, and properly seasoned lean proteins often work well in the night shift environment. Avoid dishes that become soggy or unpalatable when reheated, as this can lead to food waste and reliance on less healthy alternatives.

Temperature control becomes crucial when preparing meals for night shifts. Invest in a high quality insulated lunch bag and ice packs to maintain food safety throughout your shift. Consider preparing some items that can be stored in the freezer and moved to the refrigerator as needed throughout your work week. This approach provides flexibility while ensuring you always have access to properly prepared meals.

Batch cooking serves as a cornerstone of successful night shift meal prep. Focus on versatile ingredients that can be mixed and matched to create different meals throughout the week. For example, grilled chicken breast can be used in salads, wraps, or grain bowls. Roasted vegetables can serve as side dishes or be incorporated into main dishes. This approach provides variety while maximizing your meal prep efficiency.

Proper portioning plays a vital role in night shift meal prep success. Package meals in individual portions that align with your energy needs and eating schedule. This prevents overeating during shifts and ensures you maintain consistent energy levels throughout your work hours. Consider preparing slightly smaller portions for the challenging early morning hours when digestion naturally slows.

Snack preparation deserves special attention in your meal prep routine. Prepare portion controlled, nutrient dense snacks that can easily be consumed during brief breaks. Cut vegetables, portioned nuts, and homemade energy bites provide quick fuel without the crash associated with processed snacks. Store these in easily accessible containers that can be quickly grabbed during busy shifts.

Organization becomes crucial when implementing a successful meal prep routine. Create a system for labeling and storing prepared foods that allows you to quickly identify meals and track freshness. Many night workers find success using a color coding system or clear labeling with dates and contents. This organization prevents waste and ensures you always know what foods are available.

Consider the environmental impact of your meal prep routine. Choose reusable containers and storage solutions that minimize waste while maintaining food safety. This approach not only benefits the environment but also reduces the ongoing cost of disposable storage options. Many night workers find that investing in a high quality set of reusable containers pays for itself within a few months.

Variety within your meal prep routine prevents food fatigue and maintains your commitment to healthy eating. Rotate through different recipes and meal combinations to keep your nutrition interesting and satisfying. Consider preparing a mix of hot and cold options to provide flexibility throughout your shifts. This variety helps maintain consistent healthy eating patterns even during challenging periods of your shift.

Emergency meal prep provides a safety net for unexpected situations. Prepare and freeze individual portions of balanced meals that can be easily accessed when regular meal prep isn't possible. Keep shelf stable, nutrient dense options in your work space for situations when fresh prepared foods aren't available. This backup system helps maintain consistent nutrition even during disrupted schedules.

The social aspects of meal prep can support long term success. Consider organizing meal prep sessions with other night shift workers to share the workload and maintain motivation. These sessions provide opportunities to exchange recipes and strategies while building supportive relationships with colleagues who understand the unique challenges of night shift work.

Successful meal prep for night shift workers requires ongoing evaluation and adjustment. Regularly assess what works well and what needs improvement in your routine. Pay attention to which meals maintain quality throughout your shifts and which recipes need modification. This continuous improvement approach helps refine your meal prep strategy over time.

Remember that developing an effective meal prep routine takes time and patience. Start with simple, manageable preparations and gradually expand your repertoire as you become more comfortable with the process. Focus on progress rather than perfection, understanding that any step toward better preparation supports your overall success on the night shift.

Hydration Protocols for Overnight Hours

Proper hydration serves as a cornerstone of health and performance for night shift workers, yet it remains one of the most overlooked aspects of overnight wellness. The human body's natural hydration rhythms evolved to align with daytime activity patterns, making deliberate hydration protocols essential for those working through the night.

The challenges of maintaining proper hydration during overnight hours stem from multiple factors. Our bodies naturally reduce fluid regulation efficiency during nighttime hours, while the artificial environment of most workplaces can accelerate dehydration through dry air and artificial heating or cooling systems. Additionally, the reliance on caffeine to maintain alertness often compounds hydration challenges.

Creating an effective hydration protocol begins with understanding your individual fluid needs. While the common recommendation of eight glasses of water daily provides a baseline, night shift workers typically require additional fluid intake to compensate for their altered schedule and workplace environment. A more accurate approach involves monitoring your body weight and urine color, aiming for pale yellow urine and stable body weight as indicators of proper hydration.

Timing fluid intake becomes crucial for night shift workers. Begin hydrating several hours before your shift starts, focusing on steady consumption rather than large volumes at once. This approach helps establish proper hydration without causing excessive bathroom breaks during critical work hours. During your shift, aim to consume fluids consistently rather than waiting until you feel thirsty, as thirst indicates you're already experiencing mild dehydration.

The type of fluids you consume matters significantly during overnight hours. Water serves as your primary hydration source, but electrolyte-enhanced beverages can play a valuable role, especially during longer shifts or in warm environments. Choose low or zero calorie electrolyte options to avoid unnecessary sugar intake, which can disrupt energy levels and sleep patterns.

Temperature management of beverages can support your body's natural rhythms and energy levels. Cool water typically proves most refreshing during the early portions of your shift, while room temperature water may be more appropriate during the challenging early morning hours when your body temperature naturally dips. Some workers find success alternating between warm and cool beverages to help maintain alertness.

Monitoring caffeine containing beverages becomes essential within your hydration protocol. While coffee and tea contribute to your daily fluid intake, their diuretic effects require compensation with additional water consumption. Establish a cutoff time for caffeine several hours before your planned sleep period and increase water intake during this window to support proper hydration for rest.

Food choices significantly impact hydration status during night shifts. Incorporate water rich foods such as fruits, vegetables, and broth based soups into your meal plan. These foods provide sustained hydration while delivering valuable nutrients. Conversely, limit sodium heavy processed foods which can increase fluid requirements and contribute to dehydration.

Creating environmental supports for proper hydration helps maintain consistent fluid intake during busy shifts. Keep water easily accessible in your workspace, considering both convenience and food safety regulations. Many night workers find success using marked water bottles that help track intake throughout their shift. This visual reminder supports consistent hydration while providing measurable progress.

Physical activity levels during your shift influence hydration needs. Jobs requiring significant movement or exposure to warm environments necessitate increased fluid intake. Develop specific hydration protocols for different types of shifts, accounting for varying activity levels and environmental conditions. This adaptable approach ensures proper hydration across changing work demands.

Bathroom access can present challenges for night shift workers, sometimes discouraging proper hydration. Rather than reducing fluid intake, work with supervisors to establish reasonable bathroom break protocols that support proper hydration. Many facilities have successfully implemented policies that balance worker health needs with operational requirements.

Special consideration must be given to seasonal changes in hydration needs. Summer months typically require increased fluid intake, while winter's artificial heating can create surprisingly high hydration demands. Adjust your hydration protocol seasonally, accounting for environmental conditions and workplace climate control systems.

Recovery hydration after your shift supports overall health and prepares you for quality rest. Continue steady fluid intake during your commute home, tapering consumption as you approach sleep time to minimize sleep disruption from bathroom visits. This balanced approach supports proper hydration while protecting sleep quality.

Long term health implications of proper hydration extend beyond immediate performance benefits. Consistent hydration supports kidney function, cognitive performance, and cardiovascular health. Many common health complaints among night shift workers, including headaches and fatigue, improve with proper hydration protocols.

Establishing proper hydration habits requires consistent effort and monitoring, but the benefits far outweigh the investment. Regular assessment of your hydration status through simple measures like urine color and body weight helps refine your protocol over time. Remember that individual needs vary, and successful hydration protocols should be personalized to your specific situation and work environment.

Caffeine: Your Friend and Enemy

C affeine plays a uniquely complex role in the lives of night shift workers, simultaneously serving as both an essential tool for maintaining alertness and a potential saboteur of healthy sleep patterns. Understanding how to harness caffeine's benefits while avoiding its pitfalls becomes crucial for sustainable night shift success.

The science behind caffeine's effectiveness stems from its ability to block adenosine receptors in the brain. Adenosine naturally builds up during waking hours, making us feel increasingly sleepy. By blocking these receptors, caffeine helps maintain alertness when our circadian rhythms signal it's time to sleep. However, this same mechanism can disrupt our ability to rest when our shift ends.

For night shift workers, strategic caffeine consumption requires careful timing and dosage control. The half life of caffeine typically ranges from 4 to 6 hours, meaning that half of the caffeine consumed remains in your system after this period. This makes timing crucial for those who need to sleep during daylight hours. Most experts recommend discontinuing caffeine intake at least 6 hours before planned sleep time to minimize interference with rest.

Developing an effective caffeine strategy starts with understanding your personal tolerance and sensitivity. Some individuals metabolize caffeine quickly, while others feel its effects for extended periods. Track your reactions to different amounts and timing of caffeine consumption to establish your optimal protocol. Consider factors like your age, body weight, and overall health status when determining appropriate caffeine levels.

The source of your caffeine matters significantly. Coffee provides the most commonly consumed form, but tea, energy drinks, and supplements each offer different benefits and drawbacks. Coffee typically provides the most straightforward dose control and fewer additional ingredients that might impact sleep or health. Green tea offers a more moderate caffeine content plus beneficial compounds that can support overall wellness. Energy drinks often contain additional stimulants and sugar that can complicate energy management.

Many night workers fall into the trap of using increasingly large amounts of caffeine to combat fatigue. This approach typically leads to diminishing returns as tolerance builds, while potentially creating long term sleep difficulties. Instead, develop a strategic approach that includes planned caffeine breaks to maintain sensitivity. Some workers successfully implement caffeine cycling, using higher amounts during particularly challenging shifts while reducing intake on others.

Timing your caffeine consumption to align with your body's natural rhythm helps maximize its effectiveness. The early hours of your shift, when your body naturally produces some alertness hormones, might require less caffeine support. Save higher caffeine consumption for the challenging hours between 2 AM and 4 AM, when your body's drive for sleep reaches its peak.

The relationship between caffeine and hydration requires special attention for night workers. While moderate caffeine consumption doesn't significantly dehydrate the body, higher amounts can have mild diuretic effects. Balance caffeine containing beverages with adequate water intake, especially during the latter portions of your shift when fatigue might tempt you to over rely on coffee or energy drinks.

Food interactions with caffeine can either enhance or diminish its effectiveness. Consuming caffeine with high fat or protein meals can slow its absorption, potentially providing more sustained energy but delayed onset. Combining caffeine with simple carbohydrates might provide quick energy but risk subsequent crashes. Experiment with different combinations to find what works best for your body and schedule.

Creating a pre sleep protocol that transitions away from caffeine helps protect sleep quality. Replace caffeinated beverages with herbal teas or water in the hours before bed. Some workers find success using specific drinks like tart cherry juice or chamomile tea that may support natural sleep hormone production. This transition period signals to your body that it's time to prepare for rest despite the daylight outside.

Emergency protocols for unexpected schedule changes should include modified caffeine strategies. Keep a small caffeine reserve for truly necessary situations, but avoid relying on it as your primary tool for schedule adjustments. Having alternative alertness strategies, such as light exposure, movement, and social interaction, helps reduce caffeine dependence during disruptions.

Long term health considerations should influence your caffeine approach. While moderate caffeine consumption appears safe for most individuals, excessive intake can contribute to anxiety, digestive issues, and cardiovascular concerns. Regular evaluation of your caffeine protocol helps ensure it continues serving your health rather than undermining it.

The social aspects of caffeine consumption deserve consideration in the night shift context. Coffee breaks provide valuable opportunities for connection with coworkers, but be mindful of how social consumption patterns might conflict with your optimal caffeine timing. Consider establishing alternative social rituals that don't revolve around caffeinated beverages, especially during the latter portions of your shift.

Success with caffeine management on night shift ultimately requires personalization and consistent refinement of your approach. View caffeine as one tool in your broader alertness strategy rather than your primary solution. With careful attention to timing, amount, and individual response, caffeine can support rather than hinder your night shift success.

The Night Worker's Kitchen: Setting Up for Success

Creating an efficient kitchen setup becomes especially crucial when working the night shift, as access to healthy food options dwindles during overnight hours. A well organized kitchen serves as your foundation for maintaining proper nutrition and energy levels throughout your unconventional schedule.

The first consideration in setting up your night shift kitchen involves accessibility. Arrange your kitchen to make healthy food preparation as convenient as possible during your active hours. This might mean reorganizing storage spaces to keep frequently used items within easy reach and ensuring food prep areas remain well lit without disturbing sleeping family members. Consider investing in quiet appliances like silent blenders or slow cookers that won't wake others while preparing meals during traditional sleep hours.

Food storage takes on new importance for night shift workers. While traditional meal timing often allows for daily shopping and immediate food preparation, night workers need to plan further ahead. Invest in quality storage containers that keep food fresh longer and organize your refrigerator with clear sections for different meal times. Label containers clearly with contents and dates to make quick decisions during your shift when mental energy might be lower.

Strategic placement of appliances can significantly impact your success. Position frequently used items like coffee makers or electric kettles in easily accessible locations, but consider creating a separate beverage station away from main food prep areas to minimize disruption to others during daytime sleep hours. Many night workers find success with a small refrigerator in their bedroom or home office for storing shift specific snacks and drinks.

Meal prep becomes essential for night shift success, and your kitchen should support efficient batch cooking sessions. Dedicate specific areas for chopping, cooking, and packaging meals. Consider investing in multiple cutting boards and prep containers to streamline the process. A well organized system of storage containers in various sizes helps portion control and makes grabbing meals for work effortless.

Temperature control presents unique challenges for night shift workers preparing food at unusual hours. Invest in good quality thermoses and insulated containers that maintain proper food temperatures throughout your shift. Consider how different foods hold up over time and organize your kitchen to support food safety during extended storage periods.

The freezer becomes an invaluable tool for night shift workers. Organize it with clear sections for different meal categories and invest in proper freezer storage containers that prevent freezer burn. Many night workers find success preparing and freezing individual portions of complete meals that can be easily reheated at work. Consider keeping an inventory system to track frozen meals and ensure rotation of older items.

Appliance selection takes on new importance when working nights. While a standard kitchen typically focuses on dinner prep equipment, night workers need versatile appliances that support multiple meal types. Consider investing in programmable devices that can prepare food while you sleep or work. Rice cookers with delay timers, programmable coffee makers, and slow cookers become essential tools rather than occasional conveniences.

Creating designated zones within your kitchen helps maintain organization and efficiency. Establish clear areas for breakfast foods, lunch prep, and dinner items. This organization becomes particularly important when your meal timing differs from family members.

Consider using color coded containers or labels to quickly identify your shift specific foods versus family meals.

Storage solutions need special consideration for night shift workers who often eat at nontraditional times. Invest in containers that travel well and maintain food quality during long shifts. Consider how different foods hold up under various storage conditions and organize your kitchen to support optimal food preservation. Many night workers find success with modular storage systems that can be easily rearranged as needs change.

The pantry requires careful organization to support night shift eating patterns. Stock shelf stable items that can provide quick energy during challenging shift hours. Organize snacks and shelf stable meals in easily accessible locations, but be mindful of keeping less healthy options out of immediate sight to avoid stress eating during fatigue periods.

For night workers sharing kitchen space with family members, clear communication systems become essential. Establish protocols for shared spaces and appliances. Consider using whiteboard systems or digital apps to coordinate meal planning and kitchen use. This organization helps prevent conflicts and ensures everyone's nutritional needs are met despite different schedules.

Cleaning and maintenance routines need adaptation for night shift schedules. Develop systems that allow for quiet cleanup during overnight hours without disturbing others. Consider investing in quiet dishwashers or establishing cleanup protocols that minimize noise. Maintain a regular cleaning schedule that works with your shift pattern to ensure the kitchen remains organized and functional.

Success in the night shift kitchen ultimately depends on creating systems that work with your specific schedule and needs. Regular evaluation and adjustment of your kitchen setup helps ensure it continues supporting your health goals while accommodating the unique challenges of night shift work. Remember that an organized kitchen serves as the foundation for maintaining proper nutrition and energy levels throughout your unconventional schedule.

Exercise Timing: When to Work Out

E xercise timing represents one of the most crucial yet challenging aspects of maintaining wellness on the night shift. While regular physical activity remains essential for health and energy management, the traditional rules about workout timing need significant adaptation for those working overnight hours. Understanding when to exercise can make the difference between enhancing your performance and disrupting your carefully balanced schedule.

The first consideration in timing your workouts involves your natural energy patterns during the night shift. Most night workers experience their peak alertness and energy levels during the middle of their shift, typically between 1 AM and 4 AM. However, this period often represents the busiest work hours, making it impractical for many to exercise during this optimal window. Instead, consider identifying your secondary energy peaks, which commonly occur either before your shift begins or shortly after it ends.

Working out before your shift offers several advantages. Exercise naturally increases alertness and energy levels, potentially helping you stay more focused during your upcoming work hours. Additionally, pre shift workouts can help establish a clear transition from rest to activity, similar to how morning workouts signal the start of the day for traditional schedules. Many night workers find success exercising approximately two to three hours before their shift begins, allowing time for proper recovery and meal timing.

Post shift workouts present their own benefits and challenges. While exercise can help decompress after a stressful shift, timing becomes crucial to avoid interference with sleep. The key lies in allowing enough time between exercise and your planned sleep period for your body temperature and stress hormones to return to baseline levels. Most experts recommend completing intense workouts at least three hours before your intended sleep time.

The type of exercise you choose should influence your timing decisions. High intensity workouts, which significantly elevate heart rate and body temperature, require more recovery time before sleep than lower intensity activities. Consider reserving more demanding workouts for the hours before your shift or earlier in your waking period, while choosing gentler forms of movement like stretching or light yoga for the hours closer to your sleep time.

Temperature regulation plays a crucial role in exercise timing for night workers. Your body temperature naturally drops during what would be nighttime hours, regardless of your work schedule. This can affect exercise performance and recovery. Many night workers find better results by allowing extra warm up time when exercising during these naturally cooler periods. Additionally, consider how environmental temperatures during your available workout times might impact your exercise experience.

Meal timing in relation to workouts requires careful planning for night shift workers. The traditional advice of waiting two to three hours after a large meal before exercising still applies, but fitting this window into a night shift schedule demands strategic planning. Many successful night workers coordinate their larger meals around their workout schedule, either eating their substantial "breakfast" after post sleep workouts or timing their main "dinner" after pre sleep exercise sessions.

Social considerations often influence workout timing for night shift workers. Those with families might choose to exercise during hours when children are at school or sleeping to maximize family time during overlap periods. Similarly, night workers who participate in group fitness activities might need to adjust their workout timing to align with available classes or training partners, even if these times aren't theoretically optimal for their schedule.

Seasonal changes present another factor in determining workout timing. During winter months, night workers might prefer to exercise during daylight hours to maximize natural light exposure, which can help regulate circadian rhythms. Conversely, summer heat might make indoor workouts during traditionally cooler nighttime hours more appealing. Flexibility in adjusting workout timing with seasonal changes can help maintain consistent exercise habits throughout the year.

Recovery periods between workouts take on special importance for night shift workers. The unusual schedule can impact sleep quality and hormone regulation, potentially affecting recovery time. Many night workers find success alternating between higher and lower intensity activities based on their work patterns, allowing for adequate recovery while maintaining regular movement. This might mean scheduling more intense workouts on your first day off and lighter activities before returning to work.

Consistency in workout timing helps establish routine, but night shift workers need to build flexibility into their schedule. Rotating shifts, overtime requirements, and family obligations can all necessitate adjustments to exercise timing. Developing multiple workout options for different timing scenarios helps maintain regular physical activity despite schedule variations. For example, having both a preferred workout time and a backup option ensures you can still exercise even when your primary timing window becomes unavailable.

The relationship between exercise timing and sleep quality requires careful consideration for night shift workers. While regular physical activity generally improves sleep quality, poorly timed workouts can interfere with rest. Monitor how different exercise timing affects your sleep patterns and adjust accordingly. Some workers find that morning workouts after their shift actually help them fall asleep better, while others need that time for immediate rest and prefer exercising later in their waking period.

Weather and seasonal conditions can impact optimal workout timing for night shift workers, particularly for those who enjoy outdoor exercise. Safety considerations might necessitate adjusting workout times to daylight hours, especially during winter months. Similarly, extreme weather conditions might influence when outdoor activities become practical. Maintaining flexibility in workout timing while considering these environmental factors helps ensure consistent exercise habits throughout the year.

Long term sustainability should guide your decisions about exercise timing. While the theoretically optimal workout time might occur at a certain hour, practical considerations often require compromise. The best workout timing ultimately becomes the one you can maintain consistently within your life circumstances. Regular evaluation and adjustment of your exercise schedule helps ensure it continues supporting your overall wellness goals while accommodating the unique demands of night shift work.

High-Energy Workouts for Night Shift Workers

High energy workouts serve as a vital component of maintaining physical and mental wellness while working the night shift. These intense exercise sessions can help regulate your circadian rhythm, boost alertness during work hours, and improve overall fitness despite an unconventional schedule. The key lies in selecting and modifying workouts that align with both your energy patterns and the unique demands of night shift work.

Interval training stands out as particularly effective for night shift workers, offering significant benefits in relatively short time periods. By alternating between periods of high intensity effort and active recovery, you can maximize your workout efficiency while maintaining the energy reserves needed for your shift. A basic interval protocol might involve 30 seconds of maximum effort followed by 90 seconds of lower intensity movement, repeated for 20 to 30 minutes. This approach proves especially valuable when training time feels limited by sleep and work obligations.

Circuit training provides another powerful option for night shift workers seeking high energy workouts. By combining strength exercises with cardio elements, circuits maintain elevated heart rates while building functional strength. A typical circuit might include bodyweight exercises like burpees, mountain climbers, and jump squats interspersed with resistance training movements. The continuous movement between exercises helps prevent the energy crashes that can occur during traditional strength training sessions, making it easier to transition back to work or prepare for sleep, depending on your workout timing.

High intensity resistance training offers particular benefits for night shift workers looking to maintain muscle mass and bone density, which can be compromised by irregular schedules. Instead of traditional slow paced weight lifting, focus on compound movements performed with moderate weights and minimal rest periods. This approach elevates both heart rate and metabolic rate while building strength. Exercises like deadlifts, push presses, and rowing combinations work multiple muscle groups simultaneously, maximizing workout efficiency.

Plyometric exercises can significantly boost energy levels and mental alertness when appropriately incorporated into night shift workouts. These explosive movements, including box jumps, clapping push ups, and medicine ball throws, engage fast twitch muscle fibers while stimulating the nervous system. However, proper warm up becomes especially crucial when performing plyometrics during naturally lower energy periods of your biological clock. Start with lower intensity variations and gradually progress to more demanding versions as your body adapts.

Combat sports inspired workouts provide an engaging way to maintain high energy output while developing functional fitness. Boxing, kickboxing, and martial arts movements combine cardio conditioning with strength development and stress relief. The varied nature of these workouts helps prevent boredom while challenging both body and mind. Even without specialized equipment, shadow boxing and bodyweight martial arts movements can deliver an intense workout adaptable to any schedule or location.

Metabolic conditioning workouts specifically target the energy systems most relevant to maintaining alertness and performance during night shifts. These sessions typically involve full body movements performed in carefully structured work to rest ratios. For example, kettlebell swings, battle rope waves, and sled pushes can be combined in short, intense blocks followed by brief recovery periods. This training style helps improve both aerobic and anaerobic capacity while enhancing work performance.

Dance based high intensity workouts offer a mentally engaging option that can help combat the monotony often associated with night shift schedules. Whether following structured dance fitness programs or creating your own high energy movement sequences, these workouts elevate heart rate while improving coordination and spatial awareness. The rhythmic nature of dance movement can also help maintain natural movement patterns that might otherwise become disrupted by prolonged periods of seated work.

When designing high energy workouts for the night shift, consider incorporating elements that specifically address common physical challenges of overnight work. For instance, exercises that promote thoracic mobility and shoulder stability can help counteract the effects of prolonged computer work or standing. Similarly, movements that engage the posterior chain can offset the forward rounded posture many night workers develop.

Recovery strategies become particularly important when maintaining a high energy workout routine on the night shift. While intense exercise provides numerous benefits, the unusual schedule can impact your body's natural recovery processes. Incorporate dynamic stretching, mobility work, and self myofascial release techniques between high intensity sessions. Pay special attention to sleep quality and nutrition timing to support recovery from these demanding workouts.

Adaptation periods for high energy workouts may need to be longer for night shift workers compared to those on traditional schedules. Start with shorter duration high intensity sessions and gradually increase workout length and frequency as your body adjusts. Monitor your energy levels during subsequent work shifts and sleep periods to ensure your exercise intensity supports rather than hinders your overall performance.

The social aspect of high energy workouts shouldn't be overlooked, even when working nights. Consider joining 24 hour fitness facilities that offer group classes during unconventional hours or finding workout partners with similar schedules. Virtual fitness communities can also provide motivation and accountability when in person options prove limited. The energy of group workouts, whether physical or virtual, often helps maintain intensity levels that might be difficult to achieve alone.

Remember that successful high energy workouts on the night shift require consistent monitoring and adjustment. Pay attention to how different workout styles and intensities affect your energy levels, sleep quality, and work performance. Be prepared to modify your approach based on changing shift patterns, seasonal variations, and life demands. The goal remains maintaining a sustainable, energizing fitness routine that enhances rather than depletes your capacity to thrive on the night shift.

Low-Impact Exercise Options for Recovery Days

L ow impact exercise provides an essential counterbalance to more intense training sessions while working the night shift. These gentler forms of movement allow your body to recover and adapt while still maintaining activity levels that support both physical and mental wellbeing. Understanding how to effectively incorporate low impact exercise into your schedule can help prevent burnout and injury while building sustainable fitness habits.

Walking serves as a foundational low impact exercise particularly well suited to night shift workers. Whether outdoors in quiet predawn hours or on a treadmill, walking provides cardiovascular benefits without overtaxing already stressed systems. The rhythmic nature of walking can help regulate circadian rhythms while providing time for mental processing. Many night shift workers find success in breaking up longer walks into several shorter sessions throughout their shift, perhaps using break times to accumulate movement minutes.

Swimming offers unique advantages as a low impact recovery exercise. The buoyancy of water reduces stress on joints while providing gentle resistance for maintaining muscle tone. For night shift workers with access to 24 hour pools, an early morning swim after work can serve as both exercise and relaxation. The sensory deprivation aspect of swimming can help quiet an overstimulated mind preparing for daytime sleep. Even simple water walking or treading provides beneficial movement without risking overexertion.

Yoga practice adapted for night shift schedules can provide both physical and mental benefits while remaining gentle on the body. Restorative poses help release tension accumulated during long shifts, while gentle flow sequences maintain mobility and strength. Many night shift workers find success with shorter, frequent yoga sessions rather than longer classes. Simple poses performed during quiet moments at work can help prevent stiffness, while more complete practices before sleep aid in relaxation.

Cycling on stationary bikes or recumbent equipment offers adjustable intensity levels perfect for recovery days. The controlled nature of indoor cycling allows for precise management of effort, from very light movement to moderate cardio as energy allows. This proves especially valuable when fatigue levels fluctuate due to changing shift patterns or sleep quality. The seated position reduces impact while still providing cardiovascular benefits and maintaining leg strength.

Tai Chi and Qigong movements provide gentle exercise that improves balance, coordination, and body awareness. These practices can be particularly beneficial during the natural energy lulls night shift workers experience. The deliberate, flowing movements help maintain physical activity without depleting energy reserves needed for work. Many practitioners find these exercises help manage stress while improving sleep quality when practiced before rest periods.

Pilates based exercises offer structured movement that builds core strength and stability without excessive impact. The focus on controlled movement and proper alignment helps counteract postural issues common among night shift workers. Modified Pilates exercises can be performed with minimal equipment, making them accessible during work breaks or in limited space at home. The emphasis on breathing and mind body connection provides additional stress management benefits.

Elliptical training provides a low impact alternative to running while still offering cardiovascular benefits. The smooth motion reduces joint stress while allowing for natural arm and leg coordination. Night shift workers can adjust resistance and speed to match energy levels, making this an ideal option for maintaining fitness during recovery periods. The steady state nature of elliptical work can also provide meditative benefits during otherwise chaotic schedules.

Band work and light resistance training offer ways to maintain strength without the joint stress of heavy weights. Using resistance bands or light dumbbells, exercises can focus on form and control rather than maximum effort. This approach helps prevent strength loss during recovery periods while reducing injury risk. The portable nature of resistance bands makes them particularly practical for night shift workers with varying exercise locations.

Stretching routines take on special importance as recovery exercise for night shift workers. Regular stretching helps combat the physical effects of prolonged sitting or standing common in overnight work. Dynamic stretching during work hours maintains mobility, while static stretching before sleep helps release tension. Creating a consistent stretching practice provides physical benefits while serving as a transition ritual between activities.

Balance training offers valuable low impact exercise that can be incorporated throughout the day. Simple exercises like single leg stands or heel to toe walking require minimal space or equipment while improving proprioception and stability. These exercises can be performed during quiet moments at work or as part of a more structured recovery routine. The focus required for balance work provides mental engagement without physical strain.

The key to successful low impact exercise lies in consistency rather than intensity. Regular gentle movement maintains fitness levels while allowing for recovery from more demanding sessions. Night shift workers should view these exercises as essential maintenance rather than optional extras. Building a foundation of low impact movement supports both immediate recovery and long term health goals.

Remember that recovery exercise serves multiple purposes beyond physical restoration. These gentler forms of movement provide opportunities for stress management, mental processing, and maintaining healthy sleep wake transitions. Successful night shift workers learn to value these quieter aspects of physical activity as much as more intense training sessions.

Building Strength on an Unconventional Schedule

B uilding strength while working unconventional hours presents unique challenges, but with proper planning and understanding of exercise science principles, night shift workers can make substantial progress in their strength training goals. The key lies in working with your body's adapted rhythms rather than fighting against them, while maintaining consistency in your training approach.

Traditional strength training wisdom often assumes a standard daytime schedule, but night shift workers need to adapt these principles to their reversed daily patterns. The most effective time for strength training typically falls either before your shift begins or shortly after it ends, depending on your individual energy patterns and sleep schedule. Many night shift workers find success training in the early evening before their shift, when their body temperature and hormone levels naturally peak.

Programming your strength training requires careful consideration of your recovery capacity. The stress of working nights already impacts your body's ability to repair and build muscle, so your training plan needs to account for this additional recovery demand. This often means reducing overall training volume while maintaining or slightly increasing intensity to preserve strength gains. A typical approach might involve two to three full body strength sessions per week rather than the traditional body part split routines many daytime trainers follow.

The foundation of any successful strength program lies in the fundamental movement patterns: squats, hinges, pushes, pulls, and carries. These movements form the basis of functional strength and can be scaled and modified to match your current energy levels and recovery capacity. On days when you feel particularly fatigued, focusing on technical practice with lighter weights can maintain progress while managing fatigue.

Compound exercises should form the core of your strength training program, as they provide the most efficient return on your time investment. Exercises like deadlifts, bench presses, rows, and overhead presses work multiple muscle groups simultaneously, maximizing the training effect while minimizing the time required. This efficiency becomes particularly important when balancing training with the demands of night shift work and daytime sleep requirements.

Progressive overload remains essential for strength development, but the progression may need to occur more gradually than for daytime workers. Small incremental increases in weight or volume, perhaps on a biweekly rather than weekly basis, often prove more sustainable. Tracking your progress becomes crucial, as fatigue can mask genuine strength improvements if you're not maintaining detailed records.

Recovery between sets takes on added importance for night shift workers. While traditional strength training often recommends relatively short rest periods, night shift workers may benefit from slightly longer rest intervals to ensure quality movement and maintain proper form. This approach helps manage overall fatigue while still providing sufficient stimulus for strength development.

Nutrition timing around strength training requires careful coordination with your work schedule. Pre workout nutrition should occur about two to three hours before training, which might mean eating a substantial meal at the beginning of your shift if you plan to train afterward. Post workout nutrition becomes equally important, though you'll need to balance it with your approaching sleep window if training after your shift.

The role of supplementation deserves consideration in a night shift strength training program. While whole food sources should provide the majority of your nutrients, strategic supplementation with protein, creatine, and essential minerals can help support recovery and strength development. The timing of these supplements should align with your adjusted eating and training schedule rather than following traditional recommendations.

Deload weeks take on special significance for night shift workers engaged in strength training. Planning regular periods of reduced training intensity, perhaps every fourth or fifth week, helps prevent accumulative fatigue and reduces injury risk. During these deload periods, maintaining movement through lighter training or recovery exercises helps preserve gains while allowing for fuller recovery.

Equipment selection can significantly impact training success for night shift workers. Having access to both free weights and machines provides valuable options for days when fatigue might impact coordination and balance. Safety considerations become particularly important when training during off peak hours, so having appropriate equipment and backup plans for solo training becomes essential.

Creating a sustainable strength training environment at home can provide valuable flexibility in your training schedule. Basic equipment like adjustable dumbbells, resistance bands, and a sturdy bench allow for effective strength work without requiring gym access. This setup proves especially valuable during schedule disruptions or when time constraints make gym visits impractical.

The psychological aspects of strength training on night shift deserve attention. Setting realistic expectations and acknowledging that progress might occur more slowly than for daytime trainers helps maintain motivation. Celebrating small victories and focusing on consistency rather than perfect performance helps build sustainable habits.

Monitoring your body's responses to strength training becomes crucial when working nights. Paying attention to sleep quality, recovery rates, and energy levels helps guide training decisions and prevent overreach. Learning to adjust training intensity based on these feedback signals helps maintain progress while preventing burnout.

Building strength on an unconventional schedule requires patience, consistency, and intelligent training design. By understanding how night shift work affects your recovery capacity and adapting your training approach accordingly, you can make steady progress toward your strength goals while maintaining the balance necessary for long term success.

Cardio Protocols for the Midnight Warrior

Cardiovascular fitness presents unique challenges and opportunities for night shift workers. While traditional cardio wisdom focuses on morning or evening workouts, those working overnight hours need to approach their cardio training with careful consideration of their adjusted circadian rhythms and energy patterns.

The most effective cardio sessions for night workers typically align with their body's natural energy peaks, which often occur in the early evening hours before a shift or in the morning hours after work. These windows allow for maximum effort and optimal physiological response while minimizing disruption to sleep patterns and recovery cycles.

Intensity management becomes crucial for overnight workers engaging in cardio training. High intensity interval training (HIIT) can provide significant cardiovascular benefits in shorter time periods, making it particularly valuable for those balancing the demands of night work with their fitness goals. However, timing these intense sessions requires careful planning to avoid interference with sleep quality.

Lower intensity steady state cardio serves as the foundation for many successful night shift fitness programs. Activities like walking, cycling at a moderate pace, or using an elliptical machine can be performed at various points during the day without overly taxing the system. This type of cardio proves especially valuable during the middle portions of night shifts when energy levels naturally dip.

The duration of cardio sessions often needs adjustment for night workers. While traditional recommendations might suggest 45 to 60 minute sessions, breaking this into smaller chunks throughout the day or night can prove more sustainable. For example, incorporating 15 to 20 minute sessions before, during, and after shifts can accumulate similar benefits while managing energy levels more effectively.

Heart rate monitoring takes on special significance for night shift cardio training. The body's natural cardiac rhythms adjust to overnight schedules, so using heart rate zones based on traditional daytime patterns may need modification. Personal experimentation and careful tracking help establish appropriate intensity ranges for different times in your adjusted daily cycle.

Environmental considerations play a crucial role in cardio protocol design. Indoor options like treadmills, stationary bikes, and rowing machines provide consistent, safe training environments regardless of time of day. This becomes particularly important when outdoor training might be limited by darkness or safety concerns during typical training hours.

Recovery between cardio sessions requires careful attention for night workers. The combination of physical stress from exercise and the physiological demands of night work necessitates longer recovery periods than might be needed on a traditional schedule. Planning easier sessions between more demanding workouts helps maintain consistency while preventing overtraining.

Nutrition timing around cardio workouts presents another key consideration. Fueling for cardio sessions while maintaining appropriate eating patterns for night work requires strategic planning. Light, easily digestible meals or snacks before cardio, followed by more substantial nutrition for recovery, help optimize both performance and general health.

Hydration protocols become especially important when combining cardio training with night work. The body's natural fluid regulation patterns shift with overnight schedules, making conscious hydration efforts crucial. Tracking fluid intake and planning hydration around workout sessions helps maintain performance and recovery.

Cross training approaches often work well for night shift cardio programs. Incorporating various forms of cardiovascular exercise like swimming, cycling, running, and rowing helps maintain motivation while reducing repetitive stress on the body. This variety also provides backup options when preferred training methods might not be available during off hours.

The social aspects of cardio training can be leveraged to enhance consistency and motivation. Finding training partners with similar schedules, joining 24 hour facilities, or participating in virtual training groups helps create accountability and support. These connections prove particularly valuable in maintaining long term adherence to cardio protocols.

Weather and seasonal considerations require additional planning for outdoor cardio training. Night workers often need to adjust their training environments based on available daylight and weather conditions. Having indoor alternatives and flexible scheduling options helps maintain consistency when environmental factors prove challenging.

Progress monitoring becomes essential for maintaining motivation and ensuring appropriate training adaptations. Regular assessments of cardiovascular fitness, using metrics like heart rate recovery, perceived exertion, and performance markers, help guide program adjustments and demonstrate improvements over time.

The psychological benefits of cardio training take on special significance for night workers. Regular cardiovascular exercise can help manage stress, improve mood, and enhance sleep quality. These benefits prove particularly valuable when dealing with the unique challenges of overnight work schedules.

Equipment selection and availability play crucial roles in successful cardio programming. Having access to appropriate training tools, whether at home, at work, or in fitness facilities, ensures consistent training opportunities. Investment in basic cardio equipment for home use often proves valuable for maintaining program consistency.

Long term sustainability requires finding the right balance between challenge and recovery. While improving cardiovascular fitness remains the goal, managing fatigue and maintaining overall health take precedence. Regular assessment and adjustment of cardio protocols helps ensure continued progress without compromising work performance or general wellbeing.

Sleep Engineering Basics

S leep remains one of the most critical factors in maintaining health and performance for night shift workers. Understanding the fundamental principles of sleep engineering allows you to take control of your rest periods and optimize your recovery, even when sleeping during daylight hours.

The human body naturally produces melatonin in response to darkness, signaling that it's time to sleep. For night workers, this natural process needs careful manipulation to align with daytime sleep schedules. This starts with understanding your individual sleep requirements, which typically range between seven and nine hours for most adults. However, night workers often need to plan for slightly longer sleep periods to account for the challenges of daytime rest.

Quality of sleep becomes particularly important when sleeping during non traditional hours. Sleep cycles consist of different stages, each serving specific restorative functions. Deep sleep, which occurs primarily during the first half of your sleep period, provides physical restoration. REM sleep, more prevalent in the latter portion, supports cognitive function and emotional wellbeing. Night workers need to ensure they're getting adequate amounts of both by allowing sufficient time for complete sleep cycles.

Temperature regulation plays a crucial role in sleep engineering. The body naturally cools during sleep, with optimal sleeping temperatures typically ranging between 60 and 67 degrees Fahrenheit. Night workers often need to actively manage room temperature during daylight hours when ambient temperatures tend to be higher. This might involve using air conditioning, fans, or other cooling methods to create ideal sleeping conditions.

The timing of sleep for night workers requires careful consideration. Most successful night shift workers find that sleeping immediately after their shift provides the most restorative rest. This approach minimizes exposure to daylight before sleep and allows the body to take advantage of natural fatigue following work. However, some individuals find success with splitting their sleep into two shorter periods, though this requires careful management to ensure adequate total sleep time.

Creating a consistent pre sleep routine helps signal to your body that it's time to rest, regardless of external cues. This might include activities like gentle stretching, reading, or meditation. The key lies in consistency, performing the same activities in the same order before each sleep period. This helps establish a conditioned response, making it easier to fall asleep even when your body's natural rhythms suggest otherwise.

Sleep debt accumulates when we consistently get less sleep than our bodies require. Night workers are particularly vulnerable to sleep debt due to the challenges of daytime sleeping and social obligations that might interrupt rest periods. Understanding and tracking sleep debt allows for proactive management through strategic napping and occasional extended sleep periods during days off.

Environmental control becomes paramount in sleep engineering for night workers. Light exposure, noise levels, and physical comfort all influence sleep quality. Creating a sleep sanctuary that addresses these factors often requires investment in specific equipment and modifications to your sleeping space. This might include blackout curtains, white noise machines, supportive bedding, and other tools designed to optimize sleep conditions.

The role of exercise in sleep engineering cannot be overlooked. Physical activity influences sleep quality, but timing becomes crucial for night workers. Moderate exercise during work hours can help maintain alertness, while avoiding intense exercise too close to bedtime prevents sleep disruption. Finding the right balance and timing of physical activity supports both performance and rest.

Nutrition plays a significant role in sleep quality. Night workers need to carefully manage their eating patterns to support good sleep. Heavy meals close to sleep time can disrupt rest, while going to bed hungry can also interfere with sleep quality. Light, easily digestible foods consumed at appropriate intervals help maintain both energy levels during work and sleep quality during rest periods.

Caffeine management becomes particularly important in sleep engineering for night workers. While caffeine helps maintain alertness during shifts, its long half life means consumption needs careful timing to avoid interference with sleep. Most successful night workers establish strict cutoff times for caffeine consumption, typically several hours before their planned sleep period.

The psychological aspects of sleep engineering deserve special attention. Anxiety about getting enough sleep often creates a self fulfilling prophecy of poor rest. Developing mental strategies to manage sleep related stress, such as relaxation techniques and cognitive reframing, helps prevent this common challenge. Accepting that daytime sleep patterns might differ from traditional night sleep while still providing adequate rest helps reduce sleep related anxiety.

Recovery from sleep disruptions requires specific strategies for night workers. When unavoidable interruptions occur, having established protocols for returning to sleep helps minimize the impact on overall rest quality. This might include relaxation techniques, brief physical activity, or light therapy, depending on the timing and nature of the disruption.

Tracking sleep patterns provides valuable insights for optimizing rest quality. Many night workers benefit from maintaining sleep logs or using sleep tracking devices to monitor their rest patterns. This data helps identify both successful strategies and areas needing improvement in sleep engineering efforts.

The social aspects of sleep engineering often present significant challenges for night workers. Communication with family, friends, and service providers about your sleep schedule helps prevent unnecessary interruptions. Establishing clear boundaries around sleep time while maintaining flexibility for important events helps balance social needs with sleep requirements.

Long term success in sleep engineering requires regular assessment and adjustment of strategies. As seasons change, work demands shift, and life circumstances evolve, sleep needs and challenges may change. Regular review and refinement of sleep protocols helps maintain optimal rest quality over time.

Remember that sleep engineering represents an ongoing process rather than a one time solution. Successful night workers continually refine their approach based on experience and changing circumstances. While the principles remain constant, individual application requires personalization and adaptation over time.

Creating Your Perfect Sleep Environment

C reating the optimal sleep environment is essential for night shift workers who need to get quality rest during daylight hours. Your bedroom should be transformed into a sanctuary specifically designed to support daytime sleep, with careful attention paid to every environmental factor that could impact your rest.

Light control stands as the most critical element in designing your sleep space. Natural daylight serves as one of the strongest signals to our circadian rhythm, so eliminating it completely from your bedroom during sleep hours is crucial. Start with installing blackout curtains or shades that are specifically designed to block 100% of incoming light. Look for options that seal tightly against the window frame to prevent light leakage around the edges. For maximum effectiveness, consider using a double-layer approach: blackout curtains paired with light-blocking cellular shades.

Temperature control comes next in importance. The ideal sleeping temperature falls between 60 and 67 degrees Fahrenheit, but maintaining this range during daylight hours often requires more effort than nighttime sleeping. Consider installing a separate temperature control unit for your bedroom if your home's cooling system struggles to maintain consistent temperatures during the day. Ceiling fans can help circulate air and create a cooling effect without dramatically increasing energy costs.

Sound management requires a multifaceted approach. The challenges of daytime sleep include neighborhood noise, traffic, construction, and the general bustle of daily life. Start with basic soundproofing measures like weather stripping around doors and windows. Consider adding sound-dampening curtains or installing acoustic panels on walls. White noise machines or fans can help mask irregular outside noises that might otherwise disturb your sleep. Some night workers find success with pink noise, which contains lower frequencies and can feel more natural than traditional white noise.

Your bed itself deserves careful consideration. Invest in a high-quality mattress that supports your preferred sleep position and maintains proper spinal alignment. Consider mattresses specifically designed to regulate temperature, as sleeping during warmer daytime hours can make temperature regulation more challenging. Your choice of bedding materials also impacts sleep quality. Natural fibers like cotton and bamboo offer better breathability than synthetic materials, helping maintain optimal sleeping temperature.

Air quality plays a surprisingly important role in sleep quality. Daytime air often contains more pollutants and allergens than nighttime air, particularly in urban areas. Installing an air purifier in your bedroom helps create a cleaner sleep environment. Look for models with HEPA filters and consider those with activated carbon filters to remove odors. Keep your bedroom well-ventilated when you're not sleeping to prevent staleness.

The psychological aspects of your sleep environment deserve attention too. Your bedroom should feel separate from the rest of your living space, creating a distinct transition from wake to sleep. Consider using calming colors on walls and bedding, as certain hues can promote relaxation. Remove or cover bright electronics and clocks that might create anxiety about sleep time. Some night workers find success with aromatherapy, using lavender or other calming scents to signal sleep time.

Organization within your sleep space helps reduce mental clutter that could interfere with rest. Keep your bedroom free from work-related items or materials that might remind you of daytime responsibilities. Create dedicated storage solutions for sleep-related items like eye masks, earplugs, and any supplements you might use to support your rest. Having these items organized and easily accessible helps streamline your pre-sleep routine.

Emergency preparedness within your sleep environment requires special consideration. While you want to minimize disruptions, you also need to ensure you can respond to urgent situations. Consider installing a special phone line or notification system that only alerts you for true emergencies. Position your phone or alarm clock where you can access it quickly if needed, but not where it will create anxiety or temptation to check it during sleep hours.

Humidity control often gets overlooked but can significantly impact sleep quality. The ideal sleeping environment maintains humidity between 30% and 50%. During daytime hours, especially in warmer months, humidity can rise above comfortable levels. Consider using a dehumidifier in your bedroom if you live in a humid climate. Conversely, in very dry environments, a humidifier might help prevent the discomfort of dried nasal passages that can disrupt sleep.

Regular maintenance of your sleep environment ensures it continues to support quality rest. Establish a schedule for cleaning or replacing air filters, washing bedding, and checking the effectiveness of your light-blocking solutions. Seasonal adjustments might be necessary as daylight hours and temperatures change throughout the year. Pay attention to how environmental changes impact your sleep quality and be prepared to make adjustments as needed.

Remember that creating your perfect sleep environment is an investment in your health and performance. While some solutions might require initial expense, the long-term benefits of quality sleep far outweigh the costs. Start with the most critical elements like light and temperature control, then gradually enhance other aspects of your sleep environment as resources allow. Monitor how different changes impact your sleep quality and be willing to adjust your approach based on personal experience and changing needs.

Blackout Strategies: Making Day Feel Like Night

Creating total darkness during daylight hours presents unique challenges for night shift workers who need quality sleep. While basic blackout curtains provide a good starting point, truly optimizing your sleep environment requires a comprehensive approach to light management that addresses every possible source of unwanted illumination.

The first step in creating an effective blackout strategy involves a thorough assessment of your bedroom's light infiltration points. Beyond windows, light can enter through door frames, air vents, cable outlets, and even the smallest gaps in window frames. Conducting a daylight inspection helps identify these subtle light sources that might otherwise go unnoticed. Stand in your darkened room for several minutes, allowing your eyes to adjust, and note any visible light penetration.

Window treatment requires a multilayered approach for maximum effectiveness. While blackout curtains serve as the primary defense, they often benefit from supplementary solutions. Consider installing blackout cellular shades behind your curtains, creating a dual barrier against sunlight. The honeycomb structure of cellular shades not only blocks light but also provides additional insulation, helping maintain optimal sleep temperature. When selecting curtains, look for options with velcro sides that can attach directly to the wall, eliminating light leakage around the edges.

Door sealing often requires special attention, as standard doors typically allow significant light penetration around their frames. Installing door sweeps at the bottom and weather stripping around the sides and top can dramatically reduce light infiltration. For extreme cases, some night workers opt for installing a light-blocking curtain over their bedroom door, creating an additional barrier against hallway light.

Small light sources within the bedroom itself can undermine even the most effective window treatments. Electronic devices with LED indicators, alarm clocks, and charging stations all contribute to ambient light that can disrupt sleep. Consider covering these necessary devices with light-blocking tape or repositioning them to face away from your sleeping area. Some workers create dedicated charging stations inside drawers or closets to completely eliminate electronic light pollution.

Portable solutions prove invaluable when traveling or dealing with temporary sleeping arrangements. High-quality sleep masks designed specifically for daytime sleeping can provide additional darkness even in well-blackened rooms. Look for masks with molded eye cups that prevent pressure on your eyelids while maintaining total darkness. Some advanced models incorporate cooling materials or aromatherapy features for enhanced sleep promotion.

Seasonal variations require adjusting your blackout strategy throughout the year. Summer months bring longer daylight hours and more intense sunlight, often necessitating additional light-blocking measures. Consider installing removable window films that can provide extra protection during peak sunlight months without permanently altering your windows. These films can also help regulate temperature by reducing solar heat gain.

Light management extends beyond your immediate sleeping area. Creating a graduated darkness transition zone between your bedroom and the rest of your home can help ease the psychological adjustment between light and dark environments. Consider installing dimmer switches or using lower-wattage bulbs in adjacent hallways and bathrooms. This creates a buffer zone that helps maintain your light-sensitive state when brief awakenings are necessary.

Emergency preparedness requires balancing the need for complete darkness with safety considerations. Install small, red-tinted night lights in strategic locations to provide emergency illumination without disrupting your circadian rhythm. Red light has minimal impact on melatonin production compared to blue or white light, making it ideal for occasional nighttime navigation.

Maintenance of your blackout systems ensures their continued effectiveness. Regularly inspect curtains and shades for wear or damage that might compromise their light-blocking capabilities. Clean window tracks and ensure proper operation of all moving parts to maintain tight seals. Replace weatherstripping and door sweeps as they wear down to prevent light leakage from developing over time.

Cost considerations often influence blackout strategy implementation. While high-end solutions like motorized blackout shades or custom-fitted window coverings offer optimal performance, effective light blocking can be achieved on any budget. Start with basic blackout curtains and gradually enhance your setup as resources allow. Focus initial investments on the most problematic light sources in your space.

The psychological impact of complete darkness shouldn't be underestimated. Some night workers initially find total blackout conditions unsettling or claustrophobic. Gradually implementing your blackout strategy while maintaining some control over light levels can help ease this transition. Consider installing dimmer switches or using adjustable blackout solutions that allow you to customize the level of darkness to your comfort level.

Remember that creating effective darkness for daytime sleep represents an ongoing process rather than a one-time solution. As seasons change, schedules shift, and new light challenges emerge, your blackout strategy may require adjustment. Maintain flexibility in your approach while staying committed to the core goal of creating an environment conducive to quality daytime sleep.

Sleep Rituals and Wind-Down Routines

Creating effective sleep rituals and wind-down routines proves essential for night shift workers transitioning from work to rest during daylight hours. Unlike traditional evening routines that naturally align with the setting sun, night workers must deliberately engineer their bodies and minds for sleep when the world is awakening.

The foundation of an effective wind-down routine begins several hours before your planned sleep time. Just as traditional workers gradually decrease activity levels as evening approaches, night shift workers should begin reducing stimulation and planning their transition to rest well before heading home from work. This might mean avoiding intense workplace conversations or challenging tasks during the final hour of your shift when possible.

Consistency forms the cornerstone of an effective sleep ritual. Your brain responds to repeated patterns by beginning its sleep preparation process when it recognizes familiar cues. Establish a sequence of actions that you perform in the same order each day before sleep. This might include changing into designated sleep clothes, performing gentle stretches, or engaging in quiet activities that signal to your body that rest approaches.

Physical preparation plays a crucial role in sleep readiness. A shower or bath can serve as both a cleansing ritual and a temperature regulation tool. The natural drop in body temperature that follows a warm shower mimics the temperature decrease that typically occurs during natural nighttime sleep onset. Some workers find success with aromatherapy during their shower, using lavender or other calming scents to enhance relaxation.

Nutrition choices during your wind-down period significantly impact sleep quality. Consider having a small, sleep-promoting snack about an hour before bed. Foods containing a combination of complex carbohydrates and proteins can help maintain stable blood sugar levels during sleep. However, avoid heavy meals that might cause discomfort or require significant digestion energy.

Digital device management becomes particularly important during the wind-down period. While many night workers use technology to stay connected with family or wind down after work, the blue light emitted by screens can significantly disrupt sleep onset. Implement a strict device cutoff at least one hour before sleep, or use blue light blocking features and settings if device use proves unavoidable.

Mindfulness practices incorporated into your sleep ritual can help quiet an active mind and reduce work-related stress that might otherwise prevent sleep. Simple breathing exercises, progressive muscle relaxation, or guided meditation can create a mental transition between work and rest. These practices prove especially valuable for workers in high-stress environments like healthcare or emergency services.

Creating a sleep sanctuary involves more than just physical darkness. Temperature, sound, and comfort considerations should be addressed as part of your wind-down routine. Set your bedroom temperature slightly cool, around 65-68 degrees Fahrenheit, as your ritual begins. Address any potential noise disruptions by activating white noise machines or ensuring sound-blocking measures are in place.

Physical comfort rituals might include gentle stretching or self-massage, particularly focusing on areas that accumulate tension during work hours. Many night shift workers develop specific muscle tension patterns from their work activities. Incorporating targeted stretching or using self-massage tools during your wind-down period can help release this physical stress.

Journal writing or thought downloading often helps clear mental clutter before sleep. Rather than lying awake processing the events of your shift or worrying about upcoming responsibilities, spend a few minutes writing down any persistent thoughts, concerns, or tasks that need attention after you wake. This practice helps create mental closure for your day.

Some workers benefit from incorporating calming hobbies into their wind-down routine. Activities like reading physical books, working on puzzles, or engaging in gentle crafts can provide a peaceful transition period. Choose activities that bring genuine enjoyment without creating excitement or stress.

Family considerations often require creative adaptation of sleep rituals. If you share your living space with others who operate on traditional schedules, establish clear communication about your wind-down needs. Create signals or systems that help family members understand when you're entering your sleep preparation phase.

Flexibility within consistency remains important when establishing sleep rituals. While maintaining a regular routine supports good sleep hygiene, your wind-down process should adapt to changing circumstances without creating additional stress. Develop both ideal and abbreviated versions of your routine to accommodate unexpected schedule changes or disruptions.

The length of your wind-down routine may require experimentation to optimize. While some workers find success with brief, 15-minute routines, others need an hour or more to effectively transition to sleep. Pay attention to your body's responses and adjust your timeline accordingly.

Remember that establishing effective sleep rituals requires patience and persistence. Your body and mind need time to recognize and respond to new sleep cues. Maintain your chosen routine even when it initially feels ineffective, allowing several weeks for new habits to become established and effective.

Managing Sleep Debt

S leep debt accumulates silently but impacts night shift workers profoundly, affecting everything from cognitive performance to physical health. Understanding and managing sleep debt becomes crucial for sustaining a healthy life while working unconventional hours. Unlike traditional workers who might occasionally miss sleep, night shift workers face unique challenges in maintaining consistent sleep patterns and often accumulate sleep debt more rapidly.

Sleep debt represents the cumulative effect of not getting enough quality sleep over time. For night shift workers, this debt often builds through small daily deficits rather than dramatic single instances of sleep loss. When you consistently get six hours of sleep instead of your body's required seven or eight hours, that missing time adds up, creating a sleep deficit that your body must eventually reconcile.

The impact of sleep debt manifests in various ways, often subtle at first but increasingly noticeable over time. Cognitive effects typically appear first, with workers experiencing decreased attention spans, slower reaction times, and difficulty with complex decision-making. These changes might seem minor initially, perhaps just requiring an extra cup of coffee to overcome, but they can significantly impact both work performance and personal safety.

Physical manifestations of sleep debt often follow cognitive symptoms. Your body may experience increased inflammation, weakened immune response, and hormonal imbalances that affect everything from appetite to emotional regulation. Night shift workers frequently report weight management difficulties and digestive issues, both of which can be exacerbated by accumulated sleep debt.

Managing sleep debt requires both preventive strategies and recovery techniques. The first step involves accurate assessment of your current sleep situation. Keep a detailed sleep log for at least two weeks, recording not just the hours you spend in bed but the quality of sleep you achieve. Note interruptions, how refreshed you feel upon waking, and any factors that might have impacted your rest.

Prevention strategies start with protecting your designated sleep hours. This means treating your daytime sleep period with the same respect others give to nighttime rest. Avoid scheduling appointments or accepting commitments during your sleep window whenever possible. When interruptions prove unavoidable, develop a plan to compensate for the lost rest either before or after the disruption.

Recovery from accumulated sleep debt requires a systematic approach rather than trying to make up all lost sleep at once. Instead of attempting to sleep for extremely long periods on your days off, which can disrupt your circadian rhythm, focus on extending your regular sleep periods by small increments. Adding 30 to 60 minutes to your usual sleep time allows for gradual debt repayment while maintaining schedule consistency.

Strategic napping plays a crucial role in managing sleep debt for night workers. Rather than viewing naps as a sign of poor sleep hygiene, recognize them as a valuable tool for maintaining alertness and reducing sleep debt accumulation. Short naps of 20 to 30 minutes during breaks can help bridge the gap between longer sleep periods and prevent excessive debt buildup.

The concept of sleep banking can help night shift workers prepare for known periods of sleep disruption. When you anticipate schedule changes or unavoidable sleep loss, deliberately getting extra sleep in the days leading up to these events can create a protective buffer against fatigue. This proactive approach helps minimize the impact of occasional sleep disruptions on your overall well-being.

Understanding the difference between acute and chronic sleep debt helps in developing appropriate management strategies. Acute sleep debt, accumulated over a few days, can usually be resolved with a few good nights of sleep. Chronic sleep debt, built up over weeks or months, requires a more comprehensive recovery approach and might necessitate temporary schedule adjustments or professional intervention.

Environmental factors significantly influence sleep debt accumulation and recovery. Optimize your sleep environment to maximize the quality of the rest you do get. This means maintaining consistent temperature, darkness, and quiet during your sleep periods. Consider investing in blackout curtains, white noise machines, or other tools that help create ideal sleep conditions regardless of the time of day.

Social and family obligations often contribute to sleep debt for night shift workers. Develop clear communication strategies with family and friends about your sleep needs and schedule constraints. While some flexibility for special occasions is reasonable, regularly sacrificing sleep for social activities can lead to dangerous levels of sleep debt accumulation.

Recovery from significant sleep debt requires patience and consistency. Your body cannot repay weeks of sleep deficit in a single weekend. Instead, focus on gradually increasing sleep quality and quantity while maintaining as regular a schedule as possible. This might mean declining some social invitations or adjusting family routines to protect your sleep time during debt recovery periods.

Professional support may become necessary if sleep debt begins significantly impacting your health or work performance. Sleep specialists can help identify underlying issues contributing to sleep debt and develop personalized management strategies. They may also recommend specific interventions or schedule adjustments to better align with your body's natural rhythms.

Remember that managing sleep debt is an ongoing process rather than a one-time fix. Regular assessment of your sleep patterns and proactive adjustment of your routines helps prevent severe debt accumulation. Stay attuned to your body's signals and be willing to modify your approach as circumstances change. With careful attention and consistent effort, night shift workers can effectively manage sleep debt while maintaining both professional responsibilities and personal well-being.

Napping Strategies for Night Workers

Napping represents one of the most powerful tools available to night shift workers, yet it remains widely misunderstood and often poorly implemented. Strategic napping can help maintain alertness, improve cognitive performance, and reduce fatigue-related errors during overnight shifts. However, the timing, duration, and environment of these naps must be carefully planned to maximize their benefits while avoiding potential pitfalls.

The human body naturally experiences a dip in energy and alertness between 2 AM and 6 AM, making this period particularly challenging for night workers. A well-timed nap can help bridge this difficult period and maintain performance levels throughout the shift. Research indicates that night shift workers who incorporate planned naps into their schedules report better concentration, improved mood, and fewer safety incidents compared to those who attempt to power through their entire shift without rest.

When planning nap strategies, timing becomes crucial. The ideal window for a night shift nap typically falls between 2 AM and 4 AM, aligning with the body's natural circadian low point. However, this timing should be adjusted based on your specific shift schedule and work responsibilities. Some workers find success with a preventive nap taken before their shift begins, while others benefit more from a nap during their designated break period.

The duration of your nap matters significantly. Short naps of 10 to 20 minutes can provide immediate alertness benefits without the grogginess often associated with longer sleep periods. These power naps work well during shift breaks and can help maintain alertness through the remainder of your work hours. Longer naps of 45 to 90 minutes allow for deeper sleep cycles but require more careful timing to avoid sleep inertia interfering with work responsibilities.

Creating an appropriate environment for workplace napping presents its own challenges. While some facilities provide dedicated rest areas or quiet rooms, many workers must improvise with available spaces. Consider keeping a nap kit at work that includes items like an eye mask, earplugs, a small blanket, and a travel pillow. These tools can help create a more conducive sleep environment even in less than ideal conditions.

The concept of the "caffeine nap" has gained attention among night workers. This strategy involves consuming caffeine immediately before taking a short nap of 15-20 minutes. The timing works because caffeine takes about 20 minutes to enter your bloodstream, so you wake up just as both the refreshing effects of the nap and the stimulation from the caffeine begin to take effect. However, this technique should be used judiciously and not too late in your shift to avoid interfering with your main sleep period.

Workplace policies regarding napping vary significantly across industries and organizations. Some progressive employers recognize the safety and productivity benefits of strategic napping and provide formal break periods and facilities for rest. Others maintain strict no-sleeping policies, requiring workers to develop alternative strategies for maintaining alertness. Understanding your workplace policies and advocating for evidence-based napping protocols can help create positive change in less supportive environments.

Managing coworker perceptions about napping can present social challenges. Some may view napping as lazy or unprofessional, despite scientific evidence supporting its benefits. Address these misconceptions by sharing information about the performance and safety benefits of strategic napping. When possible, work with supervisors to establish clear guidelines that normalize planned rest periods during overnight shifts.

Different napping strategies work better for different individuals and job requirements. Emergency service workers might need to maintain immediate readiness, making very short naps more practical. Manufacturing or healthcare workers with scheduled breaks might benefit from slightly longer rest periods. Experiment with different approaches to find what works best for your situation while ensuring you can maintain appropriate alertness for your job duties.

Recovery naps serve a different purpose than maintenance naps taken during shifts. These longer rest periods, typically taken during days off or before beginning a stretch of night shifts, help reduce accumulated sleep debt and prepare your body for the demands of overnight work. Plan these recovery naps carefully to avoid disrupting your primary sleep schedule while still gaining restorative benefits.

The transition back to work after a nap requires careful management. Establish a consistent wake-up routine that helps you return to full alertness quickly. This might include exposure to bright light, light physical activity, or other alerting strategies. Allow several minutes for sleep inertia to dissipate before resuming safety-sensitive tasks.

Some night workers experience difficulty falling asleep during planned nap periods, particularly when first establishing a napping routine. Practice relaxation techniques and maintain consistent nap timing to help train your body to rest during these periods. Remember that even quiet rest without sleep provides some benefits, though not as substantial as actual sleep.

Tracking your napping patterns and their effects helps optimize your strategy over time. Keep notes about nap timing, duration, and how you feel afterward. This information helps identify the most effective approaches for your individual needs and work requirements. Regular assessment and adjustment of your napping strategy ensures continued benefits as your schedule and responsibilities evolve.

The success of any napping strategy ultimately depends on its integration into your overall sleep and wellness plan. Coordinate nap timing with your main sleep schedule, caffeine consumption, meal timing, and work responsibilities to create a sustainable approach to managing fatigue during night shifts. With careful planning and consistent implementation, strategic napping becomes a valuable tool for maintaining both performance and well-being while working overnight hours.

Dealing with Sleep Interruptions

S leep interruptions represent one of the most challenging aspects of working the night shift, as they can severely impact the quality and quantity of rest during daylight hours. While night workers often carefully plan their sleep schedules, unexpected disruptions are almost inevitable and require specific strategies to manage effectively.

The most common sleep interruptions for night shift workers come from environmental factors during daylight hours. Traffic noise, construction sounds, lawn maintenance, and even the natural brightness of day can all conspire to fragment sleep patterns. Additionally, family activities, delivery services, and phone calls can create disturbances that would be unlikely during conventional sleeping hours. Understanding these potential disruptions allows workers to develop proactive strategies for minimizing their impact.

Creating multiple layers of defense against sleep interruptions begins with physical barriers. Beyond standard blackout curtains, consider installing sound dampening materials on walls or windows. White noise machines or fans can help mask sudden environmental sounds that might otherwise cause awakening. Some workers find success with noise canceling earbuds specifically designed for sleep, though these require careful consideration of alarm reliability.

The social aspect of sleep interruptions often proves more challenging to manage than environmental factors. Well meaning friends and family members might forget about your sleep schedule, leading to unexpected visits or calls. Setting clear boundaries becomes essential, though this must be balanced with maintaining important relationships. Consider establishing specific "do not disturb" hours and communicating these clearly to your social circle. Many workers find success with automated text responses during sleep hours that remind others of their schedule.

Technology can both help and hinder sleep continuity for night shift workers. While phones and devices offer useful tools like do not disturb modes and sleep tracking apps, they can also become sources of disruption through notifications, updates, or the temptation to check messages. Developing strict protocols for technology use during sleep hours helps maintain boundaries. Some workers find success with dedicated sleep phones that only allow emergency contacts to break through do not disturb settings.

When sleep interruptions do occur, the response strategy becomes crucial. The natural instinct might be to immediately try returning to sleep, but this can lead to frustration and increased wakefulness. Instead, experts recommend following the fifteen minute rule if unable to fall back asleep quickly. This involves getting up and engaging in a quiet, non stimulating activity until sleepiness returns. The key is avoiding bright lights and screens during these periods to maintain sleep promoting conditions.

Managing sleep interruptions also requires understanding their impact on total sleep time and quality. A single brief awakening might not significantly affect overall rest, but multiple disruptions can fragment sleep cycles and reduce restorative benefits. Tracking these interruptions helps identify patterns and adjust strategies accordingly. Many workers find that certain times of day consistently present more challenges, allowing them to plan additional protective measures during these periods.

The psychological impact of anticipated interruptions can sometimes prove more disruptive than the interruptions themselves. Anxiety about potential sleep disturbances can make it harder to initially fall asleep and maintain restful sleep. Developing confidence in your ability to handle interruptions when they occur helps reduce this anticipatory stress. This might involve creating specific action plans for common disruptions or practicing relaxation techniques that can be employed when sleep is disturbed.

Recovery strategies following significantly interrupted sleep become essential for maintaining performance during subsequent shifts. While making up lost sleep hour for hour isn't usually practical, strategic napping and schedule adjustments can help mitigate the effects of poor quality rest. Some workers find success with splitting their sleep into two shorter periods when their primary sleep is disrupted, though this requires careful planning to maintain circadian rhythm stability.

Family dynamics often play a central role in sleep interruption patterns for night shift workers. Children returning from school, partners beginning their day, or household activities can all impact sleep quality. Creating family schedules that respect sleep needs while maintaining important connections requires ongoing communication and adjustment. Some families designate quiet zones or specific quiet hours to protect the night worker's rest period.

Emergency situations present unique challenges for sleep interruption management. While some disruptions can be avoided or minimized, true emergencies require immediate attention regardless of sleep needs. Developing clear criteria for what constitutes an emergency worthy of sleep interruption helps family members and emergency contacts make appropriate decisions. Having predetermined protocols for handling various types of emergencies while maintaining minimal sleep disruption can reduce stress for everyone involved.

The cumulative effects of chronic sleep interruptions can significantly impact both health and job performance. Understanding these potential consequences motivates the development and maintenance of protective strategies. Regular assessment of sleep quality and interruption patterns allows for ongoing refinement of management techniques. This might involve adjusting sleep timing, modifying environmental controls, or renegotiating social boundaries as circumstances change.

Building resilience to sleep interruptions becomes an essential skill for long term success on the night shift. This involves both practical strategies for preventing and managing disruptions and psychological techniques for maintaining emotional equilibrium when sleep is disturbed. The goal isn't to eliminate all interruptions, which would be unrealistic, but to develop effective responses that minimize their impact on overall well being and performance.

The Weekend Dilemma: To Switch or Not to Switch

The decision to switch sleep schedules on days off represents one of the most significant challenges for night shift workers. While the temptation to return to a conventional daytime schedule during weekends or off days can be strong, particularly to maintain social connections and family relationships, this practice comes with considerable physiological and psychological costs that must be carefully weighed.

The primary argument for maintaining a consistent night shift schedule, even on days off, centers on circadian rhythm stability. Our internal body clock functions best with regularity, and frequent shifts between different sleep wake patterns can lead to a state similar to perpetual jet lag. When workers switch to a day schedule on weekends, they essentially force their bodies to readjust twice each week, once at the beginning of their off days and again when returning to work. This constant readjustment can result in increased fatigue, decreased cognitive function, and various physical symptoms.

Despite these challenges, many night workers feel compelled to switch schedules during off periods to participate in family activities, maintain friendships, or attend to daytime obligations. The social pressure to conform to conventional schedules can be intense, and the desire to feel "normal" often drives workers to attempt these transitions. Understanding this reality, it becomes crucial to develop strategies that can minimize the impact of schedule switching when it becomes necessary.

For those who choose to maintain their night schedule during off days, the benefits often become apparent after the initial adjustment period. Consistent sleep patterns allow for better quality rest, more stable energy levels, and improved overall health outcomes. These workers typically report better digestion, more consistent appetite, and fewer mood fluctuations compared to those who regularly switch schedules. However, maintaining a night schedule during off days requires careful planning and strong boundary setting with family and friends.

The compromise approach, which many workers find successful, involves partial schedule adjustments during off periods. Rather than completely reversing their sleep pattern, these individuals might shift their sleep period by a few hours, allowing for some daytime activity while avoiding the extreme disruption of a complete schedule flip. This method can provide social flexibility while minimizing circadian rhythm disruption.

Social strategies become particularly important for those maintaining night schedules during off days. This might involve scheduling late afternoon activities with friends and family, finding other night shift workers for social connections, or utilizing technology to maintain relationships across different schedules. Some workers successfully create unique traditions, such as family breakfasts when they return from work, which align with their unconventional schedule while preserving important connections.

The decision to switch schedules often varies depending on the length of off time available. Workers with single days off typically find more success maintaining their night schedule, as the brief period doesn't allow for meaningful adjustment to daytime hours. Those with extended breaks, such as vacation periods, might find it more practical to transition to a day schedule, though this requires careful planning for the eventual return to night work.

Physical exercise and meal timing play crucial roles in managing schedule transitions. Workers who choose to switch schedules must pay particular attention to these factors, as they can significantly impact the body's ability to adapt to changing patterns. Strategic use of exercise can help reset circadian rhythms, while careful attention to meal timing can help minimize digestive issues during transitions.

The impact of schedule switching on mental health deserves careful consideration. The constant adjustment can create a sense of being perpetually out of sync, leading to increased stress and potential mood disorders. Workers who maintain consistent schedules often report better emotional stability and reduced anxiety, though they may face different challenges related to social isolation.

Seasonal considerations also influence the schedule switching decision. During summer months, when daylight hours are longer and social activities more frequent, the pressure to adopt daytime hours during off periods often increases. Winter months might make maintaining a night schedule easier, as shorter daylight hours and reduced social activities create fewer conflicts.

Long term career sustainability often becomes a factor in the schedule switching decision. Workers who consistently disrupt their sleep patterns may find it increasingly difficult to maintain their night shift positions over time. The cumulative effects of regular schedule switching can lead to burnout and health issues that might force career changes. This reality leads many experienced night workers to advocate for schedule consistency despite the social challenges it presents.

The role of family support cannot be overstated in successfully managing either approach. Whether choosing to maintain night hours or switch schedules, clear communication with family members about the reasons for the decision and its implications helps create understanding and cooperation. Some families develop creative solutions, such as splitting weekend activities between day and night hours, to accommodate the night worker's needs while maintaining family cohesion.

Ultimately, the decision to switch or maintain schedules during off days remains highly individual, influenced by personal circumstances, family dynamics, and physical adaptability. Success with either approach requires careful planning, strong support systems, and consistent evaluation of outcomes. Many workers find that their approach evolves over time as they better understand their bodies' responses and as life circumstances change.

Family Life on Night Shift

Chapter 27 focuses on managing family life while working the night shift. The unique challenges of maintaining strong family bonds while operating on an opposite schedule from loved ones requires careful planning, clear communication, and creative solutions that work for everyone involved.

The foundation of successful family life on the night shift begins with establishing clear expectations and boundaries. Family members need to understand that the night worker's sleep is not optional or flexible, just as day workers' sleep is protected during nighttime hours. This often requires ongoing education about the importance of uninterrupted rest and the physical demands of working overnight. Creating visual cues, such as "Do Not Disturb" signs or using light blocking curtains, can help younger family members understand when quiet time is necessary.

Communication becomes especially crucial when working opposite hours from family members. Technology can bridge the gap, with scheduled video calls during break times or text message check ins helping maintain connection throughout the day. Many night shift workers find success in leaving notes for family members before heading to work or upon returning home, creating a sense of presence even during physical absence.

Quality time takes on new meaning when working nights. Rather than focusing on traditional family dinner times, night shift workers might establish special breakfast rituals with their children before heading to bed, or create unique traditions around their days off. Some families find success in scheduling their main meal together during the worker's "lunch break," which might fall during the family's after school hours. These intentional connections help maintain family bonds despite unconventional schedules.

Household responsibilities often require creative redistribution when one partner works nights. Traditional assumptions about who handles specific tasks may need adjustment based on wake times and energy levels. Some families find success in dividing responsibilities based on timing rather than task type, with the night worker handling early morning duties before sleep and the day working partner managing afternoon and evening responsibilities.

Children present unique challenges and opportunities when adapting to a parent's night shift schedule. Age appropriate explanations about why mom or dad sleeps during the day help build understanding and cooperation. Younger children might benefit from visual schedules showing when their night working parent is available for activities. Older children can learn valuable lessons about respect, adaptation, and the importance of work ethic through their parent's dedication to an unconventional schedule.

Special occasions and holidays require advance planning and sometimes difficult compromises. Night shift workers might need to adjust their sleep schedule to attend important family events, requiring careful management of fatigue and recovery time. Some families choose to celebrate holidays on alternate days that better align with the night worker's schedule, creating their own unique traditions in the process.

Extended family relationships often face strain when working nights, as traditional family gatherings and expectations may conflict with sleep needs. Setting clear boundaries while maintaining flexibility for truly important events helps balance these competing demands. Some night workers find success in hosting family gatherings during their active hours, introducing relatives to their schedule rather than constantly adjusting to others' expectations.

Partner relationships require particular attention when working opposite schedules. Intentional planning of couple time, whether through scheduled date nights or overlapping wake hours, helps maintain emotional connection. Some couples find that having different schedules actually provides benefits, such as individual time for personal interests or more flexible childcare arrangements.

The emotional impact of missing family moments must be acknowledged and addressed. Night shift workers might miss bedtime stories, school events, or morning routines that others take for granted. Finding alternative ways to participate, such as recording video messages or planning special one on one time during available hours, helps mitigate these losses.

Managing household noise levels presents ongoing challenges, especially in smaller homes. Some families designate quiet zones or use white noise machines to minimize disruption during sleep hours. Others coordinate activities around the night worker's schedule, planning noisy tasks or outdoor play during wake hours.

Financial planning takes on additional importance when working nights, as childcare needs might increase or decrease depending on the family's schedule configuration. Some families find that having one parent work nights actually reduces childcare expenses, while others need to budget for additional support during schedule overlaps.

Creating a sustainable family life while working nights requires ongoing evaluation and adjustment. Regular family meetings to discuss what's working and what needs improvement help ensure all members feel heard and supported. Flexibility to modify approaches as children age or circumstances change allows families to maintain harmony despite unconventional schedules.

Success stories from long term night shift workers often highlight the unexpected benefits their schedule brought to family life. Some report stronger individual relationships with their children due to focused one on one time during off hours. Others find that their unusual schedule allowed them to be present for important moments they might have missed working traditional hours.

The role of the supporting partner cannot be understated in maintaining family harmony around night shift work. Their understanding and cooperation in managing household responsibilities and protecting sleep time often determines whether the arrangement succeeds long term. Regular expressions of appreciation for this support help maintain positive family dynamics despite the challenges of opposite schedules.

Maintaining Friendships Across Time Zones

Maintaining friendships while working the night shift presents unique challenges that require creativity, intentional effort, and understanding from both parties. The traditional social fabric that most friendships are built upon - shared meals, after work gatherings, weekend activities - takes on new complexity when your active hours don't align with the rest of society.

The first step in maintaining friendships across time zones is open communication about your schedule and its constraints. Many night shift workers find success in educating their friends about their unique lifestyle, helping them understand that "just staying up a little later" isn't a realistic option when you regularly work until dawn. This education process includes explaining that your 3 AM is their 3 PM - a time when you're fully alert and social, even though it might seem strange to others.

Technology becomes an essential tool for bridging the time gap. While your friends are heading to lunch, you might be winding down for bed, but a quick video call can help maintain connection. Social media and messaging apps allow for asynchronous communication, letting you engage with friends' lives even when your active hours don't overlap. Many night workers find success in maintaining group chats where they can catch up on conversations during their work hours and contribute when others are sleeping.

Planning social gatherings requires strategic thinking. Rather than trying to force yourself into traditional evening social hours, consider hosting breakfast gatherings after your shift when you're still awake and your friends are starting their day. Some night workers establish regular "sunset brunches" with friends, creating unique social traditions that work for their schedule. Weekend gatherings might need to shift earlier in the day to accommodate your sleep schedule while still allowing for meaningful interaction.

The concept of "time shifting" becomes crucial for maintaining friendships. Just as people in different time zones learn to calculate appropriate contact hours, you'll develop a mental map of when your friends are available and when you're able to connect. Some night workers find they develop stronger friendships with people in different time zones, as their active hours naturally align better with friends several hours away.

Building a social circle within the night shift community provides valuable support and understanding. Coworkers often become close friends precisely because they understand the lifestyle challenges and share similar schedules. Many cities have social groups specifically for night shift workers, creating opportunities to maintain an active social life without disrupting work patterns.

Special occasions require careful planning and sometimes difficult choices. Weddings, birthday parties, and other significant events typically occur during what would be your normal sleep hours. Developing strategies for managing these exceptions without completely disrupting your schedule becomes essential. Some workers find success in taking strategic naps before and after events, while others carefully choose which events warrant schedule adjustments.

Long distance friendships sometimes become easier to maintain when working nights. The time difference that might challenge others works in your favor, as your active hours might better align with friends in different time zones. Many night workers find they can maintain closer connections with international friends because their unusual schedule creates natural overlap times for communication.

Friend groups often need to adapt their traditional gathering patterns to include their night shift members. Some groups establish rotating schedules for get togethers, alternating between times that work for different members' schedules. Others create monthly breakfast clubs or early afternoon activities that allow night workers to participate before sleep while still being accessible to those on traditional schedules.

The emotional aspect of maintaining friendships across time zones cannot be overlooked. It's natural to feel disconnected or left out when social media fills with pictures of gatherings you couldn't attend or conversations that happened while you were sleeping. Developing resilience and finding alternative ways to stay connected helps manage these feelings without allowing them to damage friendships.

Regular check ins become crucial when face to face time is limited. Setting reminders to reach out to friends during your active hours helps maintain connections even when spontaneous interaction isn't possible. Many night workers establish regular virtual coffee dates or gaming sessions with friends, creating consistent connection points that work around schedule constraints.

The role of understanding friends becomes invaluable. Those who make the effort to remember your schedule, plan inclusive activities, and maintain connection despite time differences often become your closest allies. Nurturing these relationships and expressing appreciation for their efforts helps build stronger, more resilient friendships that can withstand the challenges of opposite schedules.

Success in maintaining friendships across time zones ultimately comes down to creativity, commitment, and clear communication. While the traditional frameworks for friendship may not apply, new patterns and traditions can emerge that support meaningful connections despite unconventional schedules. The effort required to maintain these relationships pays dividends in emotional support, social connection, and overall well being while working the night shift.

Dating and Romance on the Night Shift

D ating and romance on the night shift presents unique challenges and opportunities that require a fresh perspective on building and maintaining intimate relationships. While traditional dating scripts often revolve around evening dinners and weekend activities, night shift workers must navigate a different landscape entirely, finding creative ways to foster connection while honoring their unconventional schedule.

The dating pool for night shift workers naturally divides into two categories: those who share similar schedules and those who operate on traditional hours. Dating within the night shift community often proves easier initially, as both parties understand the lifestyle and share compatible free time. Many successful relationships bloom between coworkers or individuals working similar hours, though this requires careful consideration of professional boundaries and potential schedule changes.

Dating someone on a traditional schedule demands exceptional communication and commitment from both parties. The initial conversation about your schedule should happen early, setting clear expectations about your availability and energy patterns. Many night workers find success in being upfront about their lifestyle during dating app conversations or first dates, treating their schedule as a natural filter for finding compatible partners.

Creative date planning becomes essential when traditional evening outings conflict with your sleep schedule. Morning dates offer fresh possibilities - sunrise picnics, early museum visits, or breakfast food crawls can be incredibly romantic while fitting naturally into your post-shift hours. Some couples find success in planning "reverse dates," where traditional evening activities happen in the early morning hours, creating unique and memorable experiences.

Long-term relationships require thoughtful adaptation from both partners. Successful couples often develop a hybrid schedule for shared time, with each partner adjusting slightly to meet in the middle. This might mean the day-working partner stays up a bit later on weekends, while the night worker wakes up earlier than usual, creating precious overlapping hours for connection.

Physical intimacy requires intentional planning when schedules don't naturally align. Some couples establish regular "date mornings" instead of date nights, while others find success in scheduling intimate time during the transition periods between shifts. The key lies in prioritizing quality time over quantity, making the most of the hours you do share.

Maintaining emotional connection across different schedules demands creativity. Technology becomes a crucial tool, with couples using voice messages, video calls during breaks, or shared digital journals to stay connected when apart. Many successful night shift relationships involve elaborate note-leaving systems, allowing partners to share thoughts, feelings, and daily experiences even when their active hours don't overlap.

Holiday celebrations and special occasions often require compromise and advance planning. Some couples choose to celebrate on alternate days that better suit their schedules, creating their own traditions rather than forcing themselves into conventional timing. Others maintain flexible celebrations, perhaps opening Christmas gifts at midnight or celebrating anniversaries over breakfast rather than dinner.

The bedroom environment presents unique challenges when partners operate on different schedules. Successful couples invest in solutions like separate blankets, white noise machines, and blackout curtains to minimize sleep disruption. Some even maintain separate sleeping spaces for certain days, prioritizing quality rest while finding other ways to maintain intimacy.

Building relationships with a partner's family and friends requires additional navigation when working nights. Being transparent about your schedule and its constraints helps manage expectations for family gatherings and social events. Many couples develop a tag-team approach to social obligations, with the night-working partner attending morning events while the day-working partner handles evening commitments.

The emotional aspects of maintaining romance across different schedules cannot be overlooked. Feelings of loneliness or disconnection can arise when lying awake while your partner sleeps, or missing traditional couple activities due to work commitments. Successful couples address these feelings openly, working together to find creative solutions and ensuring both partners feel valued and supported.

Long-distance relationships sometimes prove easier for night shift workers, as the time difference that challenges others can actually create natural overlap periods for communication. Many night workers find they can maintain stronger connections with partners in different time zones because their unusual schedule creates convenient windows for interaction.

Sexual health and intimacy require special consideration when working nights. The impact of irregular schedules on hormones and energy levels can affect libido and sexual function. Successful couples maintain open dialogue about these challenges, working together to find optimal times for intimacy that align with both partners' energy cycles.

When dating someone new, the night shift schedule can actually provide unique advantages. The inability to rely on standard dating scripts forces more creativity and intentional planning, often leading to more memorable and meaningful early dating experiences. Many night workers report that their unusual schedule helps filter out less committed potential partners early, leaving those truly interested in making the relationship work.

The sustainability of romantic relationships while working nights ultimately depends on finding someone who views your schedule as an interesting challenge rather than an insurmountable obstacle. The most successful relationships involve partners who embrace the uniqueness of the situation, working together to create new traditions and patterns that honor both schedules while maintaining strong emotional and physical connections.

For those seeking romance while working the night shift, the key lies in approaching dating with flexibility, creativity, and clear communication. While the path may look different from traditional relationships, meaningful and lasting romantic connections are entirely possible with the right approach and partner. The effort required to navigate these challenges often results in stronger, more intentional relationships built on mutual understanding and commitment.

Parenting from the Night Side

B alancing parenting responsibilities with night shift work presents unique challenges, but with careful planning and intentional strategies, you can maintain strong connections with your children while protecting your health and wellbeing. The key lies in maximizing quality time during your available hours and creating consistent touchpoints that your children can depend on, even when your schedule differs from theirs.

One of the most crucial aspects of parenting from the night side is establishing predictable routines that allow you to be present for important moments in your children's lives. This might mean adjusting your sleep schedule to attend school events, sports games, or parent teacher conferences. While it's tempting to simply power through on minimal sleep, this approach isn't sustainable and can lead to burnout. Instead, plan these occasions carefully, adjusting your sleep schedule gradually in the days leading up to important events.

Communication becomes especially important when working night shift with children. Even young kids can understand that their parent works while others sleep if it's explained in age appropriate terms. Create a visual calendar showing your work and sleep schedule, using pictures for younger children or a more detailed timeline for older ones. This helps them understand when you'll be available and when you need to rest, reducing anxiety and confusion about your absence during conventional hours.

Technology can be a valuable tool for maintaining connections during your work hours. Consider recording bedtime stories that your children can listen to, or scheduling brief video calls during your breaks to say goodnight. Some parents leave notes or small surprises for their children to discover when they wake up, creating a sense of presence even during physical absence.

Meal planning takes on added importance when parenting on night shift. Prepare and portion meals in advance so your family has nutritious options readily available. Teach older children basic cooking skills and safety rules, empowering them to handle simple meal preparation when necessary. Some families find success in preparing a week's worth of dinners during your days off, ensuring everyone has access to healthy food regardless of your work schedule.

Managing school responsibilities requires particular attention. Set up a system for checking homework and reviewing school communications during your awake hours. Many night shift parents find success in dedicating time before their sleep period to help with homework or morning routines. Create a designated space for school papers and establish a clear process for handling permission slips, school forms, and other time sensitive documents.

Childcare arrangements often need creative solutions when working nights. If possible, coordinate with your partner to minimize the need for outside childcare. Single parents or those with partners who also work nontraditional hours might need to piece together a network of reliable caregivers. Build relationships with other parents in your community who might be willing to help with school pickups or activities in exchange for reciprocal support during their needs.

Holiday and special occasions require advance planning. Consider celebrating holidays on alternate days that better align with your schedule, creating your own unique family traditions. Many night shift parents find success in splitting special days into multiple celebrations, allowing for both traditional timing and special moments during their awake hours.

Self care becomes especially critical when parenting on the night shift. Guard your sleep time carefully, teaching children to respect your rest periods just as they would respect a traditional bedtime. Use white noise machines or other sleep aids to minimize disruptions from daytime household activities. Some parents find success in rotating sleep schedules with their partner to ensure someone is always alert and available for the children's needs.

Managing guilt is a common challenge for night shift parents. Remember that quality of interaction matters more than quantity of time. Focus on making your available hours count through engaged, intentional interaction with your children. Create special traditions that are unique to your schedule, such as breakfast for dinner or midnight picnics during your days off.

Adolescents present their own unique challenges and opportunities when working nights. While teenagers require less direct supervision, they still need emotional support and guidance. Use text messaging or other async communication methods to stay connected during your work hours. Some parents find that their night schedule actually creates more opportunity for deep conversations with teenagers who naturally stay up later.

Educational support requires careful coordination when working nights. Establish relationships with teachers and school administrators, explaining your schedule and preferred contact methods. Many schools now offer online portals and email communication, making it easier to stay involved in your child's education regardless of your work hours.

Emergency planning becomes especially important when working nights. Ensure your children know how to reach you and have backup contacts readily available. Create detailed emergency procedures and post them where everyone can find them. Practice these procedures regularly so children feel confident handling unexpected situations.

Building a support network of other night shift parents can provide valuable resources and understanding. Look for online communities or local groups of parents working similar schedules. These connections can offer emotional support, practical advice, and possibly even childcare sharing arrangements with others who understand the unique challenges of your schedule.

Remember that successful parenting from the night side often requires flexibility and creativity. What works for traditional schedule families may need adaptation for your situation. Be willing to experiment with different approaches until you find systems that work for your family's unique needs. Most importantly, focus on creating meaningful connections and memories with your children, regardless of when those moments occur during the 24 hour cycle.

Social Events and Special Occasions

Managing social events and special occasions presents unique challenges for night shift workers, but with proper planning and creative approaches, you can maintain an active social life while honoring your unconventional schedule. The key lies in finding balance between participating in daytime activities and protecting your essential rest periods.

Traditional social events often occur during times when night workers would normally be sleeping. Rather than automatically declining these invitations, consider developing a flexible approach that allows you to participate selectively in the most meaningful gatherings. When a special event warrants adjusting your schedule, begin making small adjustments to your sleep pattern several days in advance. This gradual transition helps minimize the impact on your body's rhythms and allows you to fully enjoy the celebration without feeling exhausted.

For weddings, graduations, and other significant life events, communicate with the hosts well in advance about your situation. Many will appreciate your circumstances and may be willing to schedule certain activities, like wedding showers or graduation parties, at times that better accommodate your schedule. When attending daytime events, plan your recovery period carefully. Consider taking an additional day off work to readjust to your normal pattern without compromising your health.

Family gatherings often require special consideration. Rather than attempting to attend every Sunday dinner or holiday celebration, work with your family to establish alternative traditions that align with your schedule. This might mean hosting breakfast gatherings instead of dinner parties, or celebrating holidays on alternate days. Many families find these unique traditions become cherished aspects of their relationships, adding special meaning to their time together.

Birthday celebrations and anniversaries can be particularly challenging. Consider splitting celebrations into multiple parts, perhaps having a quiet celebration during your normal waking hours and a larger gathering with friends and family at a more conventional time. Some night workers find success in hosting "midnight birthday parties" or other unconventional celebrations that turn their unusual schedule into a unique and memorable experience.

Holiday seasons require careful strategic planning. Rather than attempting to participate in every traditional activity, select the most meaningful events and plan your schedule around them. Create new traditions that work with your schedule, such as celebrating Christmas Eve morning instead of evening, or having Thanksgiving dinner at breakfast time. Many night workers find that breaking free from conventional timing opens up new possibilities for meaningful celebration.

When attending social events during your normal sleep hours, develop strategies to manage your energy levels. Consider taking a strategic nap before the event, limiting alcohol consumption which can further disrupt your sleep patterns, and having a clear exit strategy that allows you to leave when needed without feeling guilty. Some night workers find success in being transparent with other guests about their schedule, which often leads to greater understanding and support.

Professional networking events and work related social gatherings present their own challenges. When possible, suggest alternative timing for team building activities or client meetings that better accommodates all schedules. Many organizations are becoming more aware of the needs of night shift workers and may be willing to schedule events at varying times to ensure all employees can participate.

Dating and maintaining romantic relationships requires open communication about your schedule constraints. Be upfront about your working hours and the impact this has on your availability for traditional date activities. Consider planning dates during your active hours, introducing partners to the unique aspects of night shift life. Many couples find creative ways to connect, such as sharing meals during unconventional hours or finding activities that align with both schedules.

Managing social media and digital connections becomes increasingly important when working nights. Use these platforms to maintain connections with friends and family during your active hours, but be mindful of setting boundaries around notification times during your sleep period. Many night workers find success in using scheduled posts or delayed messaging features to maintain social presence without disrupting their rest.

Travel and vacation planning with friends requires additional coordination. When joining group trips, be clear about your need to maintain some semblance of your usual schedule to avoid complete disruption of your rhythms. Consider booking separate accommodations if needed to protect your sleep environment, and plan activities that align with your natural energy patterns.

Creating your own social opportunities during night hours can lead to meaningful connections. Look for other night shift workers in your community and organize gatherings during your shared awake times. Many cities have businesses and activities that cater to night shift workers, from 24 hour fitness centers to late night coffee shops where you can socialize during your natural waking hours.

Remember that it's okay to decline invitations when attending would compromise your health or work performance. Focus on quality over quantity in your social interactions, and work to educate friends and family about your needs and limitations. Most people will understand and appreciate your situation when you communicate clearly and consistently about your schedule constraints.

Ultimately, successful social engagement as a night shift worker requires creativity, clear communication, and careful planning. By developing strategies that work with your schedule rather than against it, you can maintain meaningful connections and create memorable experiences while protecting your essential rest periods and overall wellbeing.

Building a Night Shift Support Network

Building a supportive network is crucial for night shift workers to thrive in their unconventional lifestyle. While working opposite hours from most of society can feel isolating, cultivating meaningful connections with others who understand your schedule and challenges can make a significant difference in your overall wellbeing and career satisfaction.

The first step in building your support network is identifying potential connections within your immediate work environment. Your fellow night shift workers are natural allies who intrinsically understand the unique challenges you face. Take time to develop these relationships beyond simple workplace interactions. Consider organizing post shift meetups for breakfast, starting a night shift book club, or creating group chats where you can share experiences and advice.

Look beyond your immediate workplace to connect with other night shift workers in your community. Healthcare workers, emergency responders, hospitality professionals, and industrial workers often share similar schedules. Many cities have social media groups or meetup organizations specifically for night shift workers. These communities can provide valuable resources, friendship opportunities, and a sense of belonging in a world that often feels designed for daytime workers.

Professional organizations and unions often have specific resources and support groups for night shift workers. These organizations can provide advocacy, educational resources, and networking opportunities with others in your field who work similar hours. They may also offer workshops or conferences tailored to night shift professionals, creating valuable opportunities to expand your professional network while connecting with others who understand your lifestyle.

Online communities have become increasingly important for night shift workers seeking connection. Forums, social media groups, and professional networking sites often have active communities of night workers sharing experiences, advice, and support. These digital spaces can be particularly valuable during your working hours when many traditional support systems are unavailable. However, its important to balance online connections with real world relationships to maintain a healthy social equilibrium.

Creating a support network among healthcare providers who understand night shift work is essential. Find medical professionals, therapists, and wellness practitioners who have experience working with night shift workers or are willing to accommodate your schedule. These providers can offer targeted support for the specific health challenges that come with working nights and may be more likely to understand the importance of scheduling appointments that dont disrupt your sleep schedule.

Family support networks require special attention and cultivation. Educate your family members about the realities of night shift work and help them understand how they can best support your lifestyle. This might include establishing quiet hours during your sleep time, planning family activities during your active hours, or creating special traditions that accommodate your schedule. Many night workers find success in designating specific family members as primary contacts for emergencies during their sleep hours.

Mentorship relationships can be particularly valuable for night shift workers. Seek out experienced night workers who have successfully navigated the challenges youre facing. These mentors can provide practical advice, emotional support, and career guidance based on their own experiences. Similarly, consider becoming a mentor to newer night shift workers once youve developed effective strategies for managing the lifestyle.

Building connections with day shift colleagues requires intentional effort but can significantly improve your work experience. Establish regular communication channels to bridge the gap between shifts, perhaps through shared digital platforms or overlap meetings. These relationships can help ensure smooth workflow transitions and create allies who understand and support your role in the organization.

Support groups specifically focused on night shift challenges can provide valuable emotional and practical resources. These might include groups addressing sleep disorders, parenting on night shift, or maintaining healthy relationships while working nights. If such groups dont exist in your area, consider starting one. Many night workers find that organizing support groups not only helps others but also strengthens their own coping strategies.

Developing relationships with local businesses that operate during night hours can create practical support systems. Build rapport with staff at 24 hour grocery stores, gyms, and restaurants. These connections can make your night shift lifestyle more manageable and provide social interaction during your active hours. Some businesses may even be willing to adjust their services or hours to better accommodate night worker needs if they recognize sufficient demand.

Emergency support networks require special consideration for night shift workers. Establish clear protocols with friends, family, and neighbors for handling various types of emergencies during your sleep hours. Create backup plans for childcare, pet care, and household emergencies that might arise while youre working. Having these systems in place can significantly reduce stress and ensure you have support when needed.

Remember that building and maintaining a support network is an ongoing process that requires regular attention and nurturing. Be proactive in seeking out new connections and maintaining existing ones. Share your successes and challenges with your network, and be willing to offer support to others in return. A strong support network can make the difference between merely surviving and truly thriving on the night shift.

The most successful night shift workers often attribute their ability to sustain their lifestyle to the strength of their support networks. By intentionally building and maintaining these connections, you create a foundation that supports not only your work performance but also your overall quality of life. Take time to invest in these relationships and remember that while working nights may set you apart from the traditional schedule, you are never truly alone in your experience.

Mental Health Foundations for Night Workers

M ental health is a critical component of overall wellness for night shift workers, yet it often receives less attention than physical health concerns. The disruption of natural circadian rhythms and reduced exposure to sunlight can have profound effects on mood, cognitive function, and emotional wellbeing. Understanding and actively managing these mental health challenges is essential for long term success on the night shift.

Working against our natural biological rhythms creates unique stressors on our mental state. The human brain is wired to be alert during daylight hours and rest during darkness. When we invert this pattern, it can lead to increased stress hormones, altered neurotransmitter function, and changes in brain chemistry that affect mood regulation. Recognition of these biological challenges is the first step in developing effective coping strategies.

Sleep disruption plays a significant role in mental health for night workers. Poor quality sleep or insufficient sleep duration can amplify anxiety, decrease emotional resilience, and impair cognitive function. Establishing consistent sleep patterns and creating a supportive sleep environment becomes not just a physical health priority but a mental health imperative. The relationship between sleep and mental wellness is bidirectional each supporting or undermining the other.

Regular exposure to natural light, even when working nights, helps maintain mental equilibrium. The brain relies on light exposure to regulate mood-affecting hormones like serotonin and melatonin. Night workers should prioritize getting some natural sunlight exposure, even if brief, during their waking hours. This might mean spending time outdoors before starting your shift or after finishing work, depending on your schedule and the season.

Maintaining consistent routines becomes especially important for mental wellness when working nights. Our brains crave predictability and structure. Establishing regular patterns for meals, exercise, relaxation, and social interaction helps create a sense of normalcy and control. These routines provide anchor points throughout your day and help combat the disorientation that can come with living on an opposite schedule from most of society.

Exercise plays a crucial role in mental health maintenance for night workers. Physical activity stimulates the production of endorphins and other mood-enhancing chemicals in the brain. Regular exercise can help reduce stress, anxiety, and symptoms of depression. The timing of exercise should be carefully considered to support both mental wellness and sleep quality. Many night workers find success with moderate exercise at the beginning of their wake cycle.

Nutrition significantly impacts mental health, particularly for those working overnight hours. The brain requires a steady supply of nutrients to maintain emotional balance and cognitive function. Eating a diet rich in omega-3 fatty acids, complex carbohydrates, and essential vitamins can help support mental wellness. Avoiding excessive sugar and processed foods during night shifts can help prevent mood swings and energy crashes that affect mental state.

Social connection becomes particularly important for maintaining mental health on night shift. The potential for social isolation increases when working opposite hours from family and friends. Making deliberate efforts to maintain meaningful relationships and create new social connections with other night workers helps prevent loneliness and provides emotional support. Virtual connections can supplement face-to-face interactions during hours when traditional socializing isn't possible.

Mindfulness practices can be especially beneficial for night shift workers. Techniques like meditation, deep breathing exercises, and progressive muscle relaxation help manage stress and anxiety while promoting emotional balance. These practices can be particularly helpful during the quiet hours of night shifts when the mind might otherwise drift toward worry or negative thoughts.

Cognitive strategies play an important role in maintaining mental wellness on night shift. Reframing negative thoughts about working nights into more positive or neutral perspectives helps reduce stress and anxiety. Acknowledging the unique benefits and opportunities of night work, while accepting its challenges, creates a more balanced mental approach to the lifestyle.

Professional support should be considered a normal part of mental health maintenance for night workers. Regular check-ins with mental health professionals who understand the unique challenges of night shift work can help identify and address concerns before they become serious problems. Many employers now offer employee assistance programs that include mental health services with flexible scheduling for night workers.

Creating boundaries between work and personal life becomes especially important for mental wellness when working nights. The unusual schedule can make it tempting to let work seep into all hours, particularly when dealing with daytime commitments. Setting clear boundaries helps maintain work-life balance and prevents burnout, which can significantly impact mental health.

Seasonal changes require special attention for night shift workers' mental health. The reduced daylight hours of winter can exacerbate the challenges of limited sun exposure, potentially leading to seasonal affective disorder. Planning ahead for these seasonal changes with appropriate light therapy, vitamin D supplementation, and increased attention to mental wellness practices helps maintain emotional stability throughout the year.

The foundation of mental health for night workers rests on understanding and accepting that this lifestyle requires unique strategies and support systems. By actively managing sleep, light exposure, exercise, nutrition, social connections, and stress levels, night shift workers can maintain positive mental health while thriving in their chosen schedule. Regular assessment of mental wellness and adjustment of coping strategies ensures long term success in maintaining psychological wellbeing on the night shift.

Combating Isolation and Loneliness

L oneliness and isolation represent some of the most significant challenges faced by night shift workers. The very nature of working while others sleep creates a natural disconnect from the rhythms and routines of mainstream society. This separation can lead to feelings of being out of step with the world, but there are numerous effective strategies for maintaining connection and combating the sense of isolation that often accompanies night work.

The experience of working through the quiet hours of night while friends and family sleep can create a profound sense of separateness. This feeling is natural and common among night workers, but acknowledging these emotions is the first step toward actively managing them. Many night shift workers report that the hardest moments come during the middle hours of their shift, when the world outside seems most distant and still.

Creating meaningful connections with fellow night workers becomes essential for combating isolation. These relationships are uniquely valuable because they're built on shared experience and understanding. Fellow night workers inherently understand the challenges and lifestyle adjustments required, making them an invaluable source of support and camaraderie. Many workplaces naturally develop tight-knit communities among their night staff, but it often requires active effort to nurture these relationships beyond simple workplace interaction.

Technology offers powerful tools for maintaining connection during unconventional hours. Social media, messaging apps, and video calls can help bridge the gap between different schedules. Many night workers find success in creating online communities specifically for those working similar hours. These digital connections can provide real-time interaction and support during the overnight hours when traditional social options are limited.

Finding ways to participate in daytime social activities requires creative scheduling and careful energy management. While it's tempting to completely switch schedules on days off to join in regular social events, this approach can be unsustainable and potentially harmful to overall wellbeing. Instead, developing a balanced approach that allows for some daytime social interaction while maintaining a relatively consistent sleep schedule proves more successful for most night workers.

The workplace environment itself plays a crucial role in preventing isolation. Creating opportunities for social interaction during breaks and quiet periods can help build community among night staff. Simple activities like sharing meals, organizing group activities during downtime, or establishing regular check-ins with colleagues can transform the workplace from a potential source of isolation into a social support system.

Physical activity can serve as both a social opportunity and a mood enhancer. Group exercise classes specifically scheduled for night workers, walking groups during breaks, or shared fitness challenges can create connection while promoting physical health. Even solo exercise can help combat feelings of isolation by providing a sense of accomplishment and physical wellbeing that supports emotional resilience.

Maintaining strong family connections requires intentional effort when working nights. Regular family meetings, shared meals when possible, and creative use of technology to stay connected during work hours help preserve these essential relationships. Many night workers find success in establishing special family traditions or activities that accommodate their unique schedule while creating meaningful shared experiences.

The role of routine in combating isolation cannot be overstated. Establishing regular social commitments, even if less frequent than desired, provides anchoring points for connection. This might include weekly video calls with friends, monthly book clubs that meet at unconventional hours, or regular gaming sessions with other night workers during break times.

Community involvement can take different forms for night workers. While traditional volunteer opportunities or community events might be challenging to attend, many organizations need support during overnight hours. Finding ways to contribute to community life, even on an unusual schedule, creates meaningful connections and a sense of purpose that helps counter isolation.

Professional development and learning opportunities can also provide valuable social interaction. Online courses, professional forums, or skill-sharing groups that accommodate night schedules offer both educational benefits and opportunities for connection with others sharing similar interests and schedules.

The importance of maintaining a dedicated space for solitude and reflection should not be overlooked. While combating isolation is crucial, learning to be comfortable with quiet periods and using them constructively can transform potentially lonely hours into opportunities for personal growth and peaceful contemplation.

Seasonal considerations affect isolation management strategies. Winter months often present increased challenges for night workers due to reduced daylight hours and fewer outdoor social opportunities. Planning ahead for these periods with alternative social activities and increased focus on indoor community building helps maintain connection throughout the year.

Success in combating isolation while working nights ultimately depends on building a multifaceted approach that combines workplace connections, family relationships, technology-enabled communication, and community involvement. By actively managing these various aspects of social connection, night shift workers can create a rich and fulfilling social life that supports their chosen schedule while maintaining essential human connections.

Seasonal Affective Disorder Strategies

Seasonal Affective Disorder (SAD) presents unique challenges for night shift workers who already face disrupted circadian rhythms and limited exposure to natural sunlight. The combination of working through the night and sleeping during daylight hours can amplify the effects of SAD, making it essential for night workers to develop comprehensive strategies for managing this condition.

The relationship between night work and SAD stems from the reduced exposure to natural light, which plays a crucial role in regulating our mood and internal clock. During winter months, when daylight hours are already limited, night shift workers may go days with minimal sunlight exposure. This can lead to a cascade of physiological and psychological effects, including changes in melatonin production, decreased vitamin D levels, and alterations in serotonin regulation.

Understanding the timing of light exposure becomes critical for night shift workers managing SAD. Strategic exposure to bright light, particularly during the early hours of their shift, can help regulate circadian rhythms and improve mood. However, timing is crucial as improper light exposure can further disrupt sleep patterns and exacerbate symptoms. Many night workers find success in using light therapy boxes during their first few hours awake, simulating the natural dawn that their schedule causes them to miss.

Creating an artificial daylight environment during work hours can help combat SAD symptoms. This involves more than just bright overhead lights. The quality and spectrum of light matter significantly. Full spectrum lights that mimic natural sunlight can be installed in work areas and break rooms, providing some of the beneficial effects of sunlight exposure even during night hours.

Vitamin D supplementation often becomes necessary for night shift workers, particularly during winter months. Regular blood tests can help monitor vitamin D levels, allowing for appropriate supplementation under medical supervision. Some night workers find success in scheduling brief outdoor time during twilight hours, maximizing their exposure to natural light while maintaining their sleep schedule.

Exercise plays a particularly important role in managing SAD for night shift workers. Physical activity can help boost mood and energy levels, but timing becomes crucial. Many find success in exercising shortly after waking, using this activity as a way to energize themselves for their upcoming shift while also potentially catching some natural light if the timing aligns with dawn or dusk.

Nutrition strategies specific to SAD management need to be integrated into the already specialized dietary needs of night workers. Foods rich in omega3 fatty acids, vitamin D, and those that support serotonin production become particularly important during winter months. Meal timing should be structured to support both energy levels during work hours and proper sleep during daylight hours.

The winter months often bring additional challenges related to social isolation, which can compound SAD symptoms. Creating opportunities for social interaction during work hours becomes even more important during this time. Many night shift workers find success in organizing regular social activities with colleagues during breaks or establishing virtual connections with other night workers facing similar challenges.

Environmental modifications at home can help manage SAD symptoms during sleep hours. While blackout curtains remain essential for daytime sleep, incorporating programmable lighting systems that gradually brighten toward the end of sleep periods can help create a more natural wake cycle. Some night workers find success with dawn simulation alarms that slowly increase light levels to mimic sunrise, even when sleeping during daylight hours.

Developing a winter wellness routine becomes crucial for night shift workers managing SAD. This might include regular outdoor activities during twilight hours, increased focus on indoor exercise options, and careful attention to maintaining social connections despite the challenges of shorter days and inclement weather. Many find success in winter specific hobbies that can be enjoyed during their active hours, such as indoor gardening with grow lights or creative projects that bring light and color into their environment.

Monitoring SAD symptoms becomes particularly important for night shift workers, as the unusual schedule can mask early warning signs. Keeping a mood journal or using mood tracking apps can help identify patterns and trigger points, allowing for proactive management strategies. Regular check ins with healthcare providers who understand the unique challenges of night work can provide additional support and guidance in managing SAD symptoms.

The intersection of SAD and shift work disorder requires careful attention and often specialized treatment approaches. Working with healthcare providers who understand both conditions helps develop comprehensive management strategies that address the overlapping symptoms while accounting for the practical constraints of night work schedules.

Planning for seasonal transitions becomes an important part of SAD management for night workers. As days begin to shorten in autumn, implementing management strategies before symptoms become severe can help maintain stability throughout the winter months. Similarly, gradual adjustments to light exposure and activity patterns as spring approaches can help smooth the transition to longer days.

Success in managing SAD while working nights ultimately requires a personalized approach that takes into account individual circadian patterns, work schedules, and lifestyle factors. By combining appropriate light therapy, physical activity, nutrition, and social support strategies, night shift workers can effectively manage SAD symptoms while maintaining their chosen schedule.

Stress Management for Night Workers

Working the night shift introduces unique stressors that can impact both physical and mental wellbeing. The unconventional schedule, disrupted circadian rhythms, and challenges in maintaining work-life balance create a perfect storm of potential stress triggers that require specific management strategies tailored to overnight work.

One of the primary sources of stress for night shift workers stems from the constant battle against the body's natural rhythms. This physiological stress manifests in various ways, from difficulty maintaining alertness during work hours to challenges getting quality sleep during the day. Understanding this underlying physiological stress helps in developing effective management strategies that work with, rather than against, the body's natural tendencies.

Creating a structured routine becomes paramount in managing stress levels. This extends beyond just sleep schedules to encompass all aspects of daily life. Successful night workers often establish clear boundaries between work time, personal time, and sleep time. This might mean setting specific hours for family interactions, maintaining a consistent exercise schedule, and creating dedicated time for relaxation and self-care activities.

Physical activity plays a crucial role in stress management for night shift workers, but timing becomes essential. Exercise can serve as both a stress reliever and an energy booster when properly timed. Many night workers find success in scheduling their workouts either before their shift to increase alertness or after work to help transition into their rest period. The key lies in finding a consistent time that works with individual schedules and energy patterns.

Mindfulness practices take on special significance for night shift workers. Traditional meditation and relaxation techniques may need to be adapted to accommodate unusual schedules, but their benefits remain crucial. Some workers find success in incorporating brief mindfulness exercises during break periods, using these moments to center themselves and manage stress accumulation throughout their shift.

Nutrition plays a vital role in stress management, particularly during overnight hours when food choices might be limited. Planning meals and snacks that support stable blood sugar and energy levels helps prevent the additional stress of hunger or energy crashes during shifts. Many night workers find success in preparing nutrient-dense meals that can be easily consumed during work hours while avoiding heavy foods that might induce sluggishness.

Social support becomes especially important in managing stress for night shift workers. Building connections with other night workers who understand the unique challenges of the schedule can provide valuable emotional support and practical advice. Many find success in creating informal support networks within their workplace or connecting with other night workers through online communities dedicated to overnight work.

Environmental modifications can significantly impact stress levels during both work and rest periods. Creating optimal conditions for daytime sleep, including proper light control and sound management, helps ensure quality rest that builds resilience against stress. Similarly, maintaining a comfortable and well-lit work environment during overnight hours can help manage stress levels during shifts.

Time management takes on new importance for night shift workers managing stress. The unusual schedule often requires careful planning to accommodate daytime appointments, family obligations, and personal needs. Successful night workers develop systems for efficiently handling these responsibilities without sacrificing necessary rest time, often utilizing digital tools and careful scheduling to maintain balance.

Developing effective communication strategies with family, friends, and daytime colleagues helps reduce the stress of maintaining relationships across different schedules. This might include setting clear boundaries around sleep time, establishing regular check-in routines, and finding creative ways to maintain connections despite conflicting schedules.

Professional development and career advancement can become additional sources of stress for night workers who might feel disconnected from daytime opportunities. Addressing these concerns through proactive career planning and maintaining regular communication with supervisors helps manage work-related stress while ensuring continued professional growth.

Regular health monitoring becomes essential in managing stress levels over the long term. Night shift workers benefit from establishing relationships with healthcare providers who understand the unique challenges of their schedule and can provide appropriate support and intervention when needed. This might include regular check-ups, stress level assessments, and adjustments to management strategies as needed.

Emergency stress management protocols become important tools for handling unexpected situations that arise during overnight hours when traditional support systems might be unavailable. Having predetermined strategies for managing acute stress, whether work-related or personal, helps maintain stability during challenging situations.

The cumulative effects of night shift stress require ongoing attention to prevention and management strategies. Successful night workers often develop personalized stress management toolkits that combine multiple approaches, from physical activity and nutrition to mindfulness and social support. Regular evaluation and adjustment of these strategies ensures their continued effectiveness as circumstances change over time.

Long term success in managing night shift stress ultimately depends on creating sustainable practices that can be maintained consistently over time. This might mean making gradual adjustments to routines, regularly reassessing stress management strategies, and remaining flexible in adapting approaches as needs change. By developing comprehensive stress management practices specifically tailored to the night shift lifestyle, workers can maintain their wellbeing while continuing to thrive in their chosen schedule.

Anxiety and Depression Prevention

Anxiety and depression present unique challenges for night shift workers due to their unconventional schedules and disrupted circadian rhythms. The combination of working against natural light cycles, potential social isolation, and irregular sleep patterns can create conditions that increase vulnerability to these mental health concerns. However, with proper preventive strategies and awareness, night workers can maintain robust mental wellness.

Understanding the biological basis of mood regulation helps in developing effective prevention strategies. The body's natural production of serotonin and other mood-regulating neurotransmitters is influenced by both light exposure and circadian rhythms. Night workers must actively compensate for these disruptions through intentional lifestyle modifications and environmental adjustments.

Regular exposure to natural light during wake hours becomes crucial in preventing mood disorders. Many successful night workers make a point of spending time outdoors before their shift begins, often combining this with physical activity. This practice helps regulate both circadian rhythms and mood-stabilizing hormones, providing a foundation for emotional wellbeing.

Creating consistent routines that support emotional stability is essential. This includes maintaining regular sleep and wake times, even on days off, to prevent the disruption of circadian rhythms that can trigger mood changes. Establishing predictable patterns for meals, exercise, and social interactions provides the structure necessary for maintaining mental wellness.

Physical activity serves as a powerful preventive tool against both anxiety and depression. Exercise stimulates the production of endorphins and other natural mood elevators, while also providing an outlet for stress and tension. Night workers should aim to incorporate regular movement into their schedule, whether through formal workouts or active breaks during shifts.

Nutrition plays a vital role in mood regulation and mental health maintenance. A diet rich in omega-3 fatty acids, complex carbohydrates, and essential nutrients supports brain health and emotional stability. Night workers should focus on maintaining stable blood sugar levels through balanced meals and snacks, as blood sugar fluctuations can impact mood and anxiety levels.

Social connections require special attention for night shift workers. Maintaining relationships despite schedule differences helps prevent the isolation that can contribute to depression. Successful strategies include scheduling regular video calls with family, participating in online communities for night workers, and finding creative ways to stay connected with friends during overlapping wake hours.

Mindfulness practices become especially important in preventing anxiety and depression. Regular meditation, deep breathing exercises, or other relaxation techniques help maintain emotional balance and reduce stress. Many night workers incorporate brief mindfulness practices during work breaks or as part of their pre-sleep routine.

Environmental modifications can significantly impact mood regulation. Proper lighting during work hours, including exposure to bright light at strategic times, helps maintain alertness and mood stability. Similarly, creating a completely dark sleep environment during day rest periods supports both quality sleep and emotional wellbeing.

Regular self-assessment becomes crucial in identifying early warning signs of anxiety or depression. Night workers should maintain awareness of their emotional state and note any persistent changes in mood, energy levels, or sleep patterns. Early recognition of concerning symptoms allows for prompt intervention before issues become severe.

Professional support plays an important role in prevention strategies. Establishing a relationship with a mental health professional who understands the unique challenges of night work provides valuable resources for maintaining emotional wellness. Regular check-ins, even when feeling well, help ensure continuity of care and early intervention when needed.

Developing strong coping mechanisms specific to night work challenges helps prevent the development of anxiety and depression. This might include techniques for managing daytime sleep disruptions, strategies for handling social isolation, and methods for maintaining work-life balance despite unconventional hours.

Building a support network of fellow night workers provides both practical and emotional benefits. Sharing experiences and strategies with others who understand the unique challenges of overnight work helps normalize experiences and provides valuable peer support. Many find success in creating or joining support groups specifically for night shift workers.

Stress management becomes particularly important in preventing mood disorders. Night workers should develop comprehensive stress reduction strategies that address both work-related and personal stressors. This might include regular exercise, time management techniques, and establishing clear boundaries between work and personal life.

Long term prevention of anxiety and depression requires ongoing attention to mental wellness practices. Successful night workers often develop personalized wellness plans that combine multiple approaches, regularly evaluating and adjusting strategies as needed. This proactive approach helps maintain emotional stability while thriving in the night shift lifestyle.

The role of sleep quality cannot be overstated in preventing mood disorders. Maintaining consistent, high-quality sleep despite daytime rest periods requires careful attention to sleep hygiene and environmental controls. Poor sleep quality can quickly impact emotional wellbeing, making sleep maintenance a crucial component of prevention strategies.

Regular engagement in enjoyable activities and hobbies helps maintain positive mood and prevent depression. Night workers should actively schedule time for activities that bring joy and satisfaction, whether during their awake hours or during overlap times with family and friends. This positive engagement provides emotional resilience and helps maintain work-life balance.

Creating Mental Wellness Routines

Creating effective mental wellness routines stands as a cornerstone of success for night shift workers. While many traditional wellness practices focus on daytime schedules, night workers must craft unique approaches that align with their unconventional hours while still delivering powerful mental health benefits.

The foundation of any mental wellness routine begins with consistency. Just as our bodies respond to regular sleep and meal schedules, our minds thrive on predictable patterns of self care and mental maintenance. For night shift workers, this means establishing fixed times for wellness activities that complement their work schedule rather than compete with it.

A comprehensive mental wellness routine typically starts with the transition into the work shift. Many successful night workers begin their "day" with a brief meditation or mindfulness practice, setting a positive tone for the hours ahead. This might involve ten minutes of guided meditation, breathing exercises, or simple quiet reflection. The key lies not in the specific practice but in its regular execution.

Throughout the work shift, micro wellness practices become essential components of mental health maintenance. These might include five minute breathing breaks every few hours, brief stretching sessions, or moments of mindful awareness while performing routine tasks. These small but consistent practices help maintain mental equilibrium during the long overnight hours.

Journaling emerges as a powerful tool for night shift mental wellness, particularly when incorporated into regular break periods. Many workers find success in maintaining a dedicated journal for processing thoughts, tracking mood patterns, and reflecting on daily experiences. This practice not only provides emotional release but also helps identify patterns that might affect mental wellbeing.

Physical movement must be intentionally woven into mental wellness routines, as the body mind connection plays a crucial role in emotional stability. This might involve scheduled walking breaks during shifts, gentle stretching sessions before sleep, or more vigorous exercise at strategic points in the day. The key lies in making movement a non negotiable part of the daily routine rather than an occasional addition.

Social connection routines require particular attention for night workers. Successful practitioners often schedule regular check ins with family or friends at consistent times, whether through brief phone calls, text messages, or video chats. These connections, while brief, provide essential emotional anchoring points throughout the week.

End of shift routines play a vital role in mental wellness, helping create a clear transition from work to personal time. This might involve a dedicated wind down period, perhaps including gentle stretching, light reading, or relaxation exercises. These routines signal to both body and mind that the work period is complete and rest approaches.

Creating space for creative expression within daily routines supports emotional wellbeing. Whether through art, music, writing, or other creative pursuits, regular engagement in creative activities provides both emotional outlet and personal fulfillment. Many night workers schedule short creative sessions during quiet periods of their shifts or as part of their wind down routine.

Mindful eating practices should be incorporated into wellness routines, as nutrition significantly impacts mental health. This involves not just choosing healthy foods but also creating mindful eating rituals, taking time to fully experience and appreciate meals rather than rushing through them during busy shifts.

Regular exposure to natural elements becomes an important component of mental wellness routines. This might involve spending time outdoors before shifts begin, maintaining indoor plants in work spaces, or using nature sounds during relaxation periods. These connections to natural elements help ground emotional experiences and provide sensory variety during long indoor shifts.

Technology management must be addressed within wellness routines, as screen time can significantly impact mental health. Successful practitioners often establish specific periods for checking social media or news, while maintaining technology free zones during certain hours. This helps prevent the anxiety and stress that can come from constant connectivity.

Gratitude practices, when incorporated into daily routines, provide powerful support for mental wellbeing. Many night workers maintain gratitude journals or incorporate gratitude reflection into their regular meditation practices. These positive focus points help maintain emotional balance during challenging shifts.

Self care rituals should be established as non negotiable components of daily routines. These might include skincare routines, relaxation practices, or personal grooming rituals that help maintain a sense of normalcy and self worth despite unconventional hours.

Regular assessment and adjustment of wellness routines ensures their continued effectiveness. Successful practitioners often schedule monthly reviews of their wellness practices, evaluating what works well and what needs modification. This ongoing refinement helps maintain the relevance and impact of wellness routines over time.

The implementation of mental wellness routines requires patience and persistence. Many night workers find success in gradually building their routine, adding new elements slowly while ensuring each addition becomes firmly established before incorporating others. This measured approach helps create sustainable practices that provide long term benefits rather than short term solutions.

Light Therapy and Mood Management

L ight therapy and mood management represent critical tools for night shift workers seeking to maintain emotional balance and regulate their circadian rhythms. The relationship between light exposure and mental wellbeing runs deep within our biology, making strategic light management essential for those working unconventional hours.

Natural light plays a fundamental role in regulating our mood and energy levels through its effects on hormone production, particularly melatonin and serotonin. For night shift workers, the challenge lies in receiving appropriate light exposure when natural patterns are disrupted by work schedules. Understanding this relationship allows workers to implement effective light therapy strategies that support both physical and emotional health.

Light therapy typically involves exposure to specific types of artificial light that mimic natural sunlight. These specialized lights, often rated at 10,000 lux or higher, can help regulate circadian rhythms and boost mood when used consistently. The timing of light therapy proves crucial for night shift workers, as improper timing can actually worsen circadian disruption rather than improve it.

Most night shift workers benefit from strategic light exposure at the beginning of their wake cycle, which typically occurs in the evening hours for those working overnight shifts. This exposure helps signal to the body that it's time to be alert and active, supporting both performance and mood. The duration of exposure typically ranges from 20 to 30 minutes, though individual needs may vary based on sensitivity and schedule requirements.

The quality of light exposure matters significantly. While many light therapy devices exist on the market, those specifically designed for circadian regulation typically provide the most benefit. These lights should be positioned at eye level or above, at a distance of about 16 to

24 inches from the face, while the user remains awake and active but not necessarily looking directly at the light source.

Beyond dedicated light therapy sessions, overall light management throughout the work shift impacts mood significantly. Many successful night workers create lighting zones within their workspaces, using brighter, bluer lights during the early portions of their shifts to maintain alertness, then transitioning to dimmer, warmer lighting as their shift progresses. This mimics the natural progression of daylight and helps maintain circadian alignment.

The relationship between light exposure and seasonal affective disorder (SAD) deserves particular attention for night shift workers. Those working overnight hours often experience limited natural light exposure during winter months, potentially exacerbating SAD symptoms. Implementing regular light therapy during these periods becomes especially crucial for maintaining emotional stability.

Modern technology offers various options for light therapy implementation. From traditional light boxes to wearable light therapy devices, workers can choose tools that best fit their specific circumstances and preferences. Some find success with dawn simulation devices that gradually increase light exposure during their wake up period, while others prefer portable light therapy lamps they can position at their workstation.

Color temperature of light plays a crucial role in mood management. Blue enriched white light, similar to morning sunlight, proves most effective for maintaining alertness and improving mood during work hours. However, transitioning to warmer color temperatures several hours before sleep helps promote natural melatonin production and better rest quality.

Creating a personal light exposure schedule requires careful attention to timing and intensity. Most successful practitioners maintain detailed records of their light exposure patterns and corresponding mood changes, allowing them to refine their approach over time. This documentation helps identify optimal exposure timing and duration for individual circumstances.

Light therapy should be integrated with other mood management strategies for maximum effectiveness. This might include regular exercise, social interaction, and proper nutrition. The synergistic effects of these various approaches often provide better results than any single strategy alone.

Environmental light management extends beyond dedicated therapy sessions. Successful night workers often modify their home environments to support healthy light exposure patterns. This might involve installing programmable smart lighting systems that automatically adjust color temperature and brightness throughout their active periods.

Regular assessment of light therapy effectiveness helps ensure ongoing benefits. Many practitioners schedule monthly reviews of their light exposure patterns and mood states, adjusting their approach based on observed results. This might involve modifying exposure timing, duration, or intensity to optimize outcomes.

The impact of artificial light on sleep quality requires careful consideration within any light therapy program. While appropriate light exposure during wake hours supports mood and alertness, excessive or poorly timed exposure can disrupt sleep patterns. Successful practitioners typically establish strict cutoff times for bright light exposure before their planned sleep period.

Understanding potential side effects of light therapy helps ensure safe and effective implementation. While generally well tolerated, some individuals may experience headaches, eye strain, or sleep disruption when beginning light therapy. Starting with shorter exposure periods and gradually increasing duration helps minimize these effects while allowing the body to adapt to the new routine.

Long term success with light therapy and mood management requires consistent application and regular adjustment based on individual response and changing seasonal conditions. Many night workers find success in creating detailed light exposure protocols that evolve with their needs while maintaining core principles of timing and intensity.

Rotating Shifts: Adapting to Change

Adapting to rotating shifts presents one of the most challenging aspects of shift work, requiring careful attention to both physical and mental wellness strategies. While some workers maintain consistent overnight schedules, many find themselves navigating variable shift patterns that can include a mix of days, evenings, and nights. Understanding how to manage these transitions effectively becomes crucial for long term health and performance.

The human body naturally resists rapid changes to its sleep wake cycle, making rotating shifts particularly demanding on our physiology. Research indicates that it typically takes the body one day to adjust to each hour of schedule change. This means that switching from a day shift to a night shift might require several days for complete adaptation. However, many rotating schedules don't allow for such gradual transitions, necessitating strategic approaches to minimize disruption.

Successful adaptation to rotating shifts begins with understanding your specific rotation pattern. Some workers face weekly changes, while others might rotate every few days or follow more complex patterns. Each schedule type requires slightly different management strategies. For instance, workers on weekly rotations often benefit from beginning their schedule adjustment a day or two before the actual shift change, gradually shifting their sleep times to ease the transition.

Sleep management becomes particularly crucial during rotation periods. Many experienced rotating shift workers develop a sleep banking strategy, ensuring they enter schedule changes well rested rather than carrying sleep debt. This might involve getting extra sleep for several days before a known schedule change, providing a buffer against the disruption to come.

Nutrition plays a vital role in managing rotating shifts effectively. The body's digestive system and metabolism function optimally on consistent patterns, making rotating shifts particularly challenging for maintaining healthy eating habits. Successful adapters often create meal plans that flex with their changing schedules while maintaining core nutritional principles. This might involve adjusting meal timing while keeping the basic composition of meals consistent to provide familiar signals to the body.

Exercise timing requires careful consideration during rotation periods. While maintaining regular physical activity supports overall health and adaptation, the timing of workouts can either help or hinder schedule adjustments. Many rotating shift workers find success with shorter, more frequent exercise sessions during transition periods, allowing for flexibility while maintaining the benefits of regular activity.

Light exposure management becomes especially critical when adapting to rotating shifts. Strategic use of bright light and darkness helps signal the body's circadian system about desired wake and sleep times. Many workers use combination approaches, employing both light therapy and light blocking techniques to support their changing schedules. This might involve using bright light exposure during the early portions of any shift to promote alertness, regardless of the natural light conditions outside.

Social and family relationships often face particular strain during rotating shifts. Successful adapters typically develop clear communication strategies with family members and friends, ensuring everyone understands the current schedule and associated limitations. Many find success in creating flexible social routines that can adapt to changing shift patterns while maintaining important connections.

Maintaining consistent daily routines despite changing shift times helps provide stability during transitions. While sleep and work times may change, keeping other activities like meals, exercise, and relaxation in relatively consistent patterns relative to wake time helps anchor the body's internal rhythms. This might mean maintaining the same sequence of activities after waking, regardless of what time that occurs.

The role of caffeine and other alertness aids requires careful management during rotation periods. While these substances can provide valuable support during adaptation, their use must be strategically timed to avoid interfering with sleep when it becomes available. Many experienced rotating shift workers develop detailed protocols for caffeine use that adjust based on their current schedule phase.

Mental preparation plays a crucial role in successful adaptation. Maintaining a positive mindset while acknowledging the challenges of rotating shifts helps workers navigate transitions more effectively. Many find success in viewing each schedule change as a temporary adjustment rather than a permanent disruption, helping reduce anxiety and stress during transitions.

Recovery periods between rotation cycles deserve special attention. When possible, building in recovery days during schedule transitions provides valuable adaptation time. These periods might involve more flexible sleep schedules and reduced commitments, allowing the body and mind to adjust more gradually to new patterns.

Environmental management strategies often prove crucial for rotating shift success. Creating sleep environments that can support rest at any time of day, maintaining consistent meal preparation capabilities, and organizing living spaces to minimize disruption from household activities all contribute to successful adaptation. Many workers develop multiple environmental configurations that they can quickly implement based on their current schedule phase.

The importance of monitoring physical and mental health during rotation periods cannot be overstated. Keeping detailed records of sleep quality, energy levels, mood, and physical symptoms helps identify patterns and potential areas for improvement in adaptation strategies. Many successful rotating shift workers maintain digital or paper journals to track these factors, allowing them to refine their approach over time.

Long term success with rotating shifts often involves developing a comprehensive approach that addresses all aspects of health and wellness while maintaining flexibility to adapt to changing schedules. This might include creating multiple versions of daily routines, maintaining various meal preparation strategies, and developing different exercise approaches that can be implemented based on current schedule demands.

Schedule Disruption Emergency Plans

L ife rarely goes according to plan, and this holds especially true for night shift workers. While establishing routines and protocols helps maintain wellness during overnight work, unexpected schedule disruptions can throw even the most prepared worker off balance. This chapter focuses on developing robust emergency plans to handle sudden schedule changes while preserving your health and wellbeing.

Schedule disruptions come in many forms. A coworker's unexpected absence might require you to extend your shift or come in early. Family emergencies could force you to handle daytime responsibilities during your normal sleep hours. Facility emergencies or natural disasters might demand all hands on deck, regardless of your usual schedule. Whatever the cause, having predetermined strategies helps minimize the impact of these disruptions.

The foundation of any schedule disruption plan starts with sleep management. When unexpected schedule changes occur, prioritizing sleep becomes crucial, even if it means taking it in smaller segments. Many experienced night workers maintain a "sleep emergency kit" containing items like an eye mask, earplugs, and perhaps some sleep supporting supplements that they can use to catch rest in less than ideal circumstances. The goal isn't necessarily to maintain your perfect sleep schedule but to prevent dangerous levels of sleep debt from accumulating.

Nutrition planning plays a vital role in managing unexpected schedule changes. Keeping shelf stable, nutritious food options readily available helps maintain healthy eating habits when normal meal timing gets disrupted. Many night workers maintain an emergency food supply both at work and at home, including items like protein bars, nuts, and dried fruits that can provide sustained energy when regular meals aren't possible. Having these options prevents resorting to vending machine fare or skipping meals entirely during schedule disruptions.

Hydration becomes particularly important during unexpected schedule changes, as stress and irregular patterns often lead to decreased fluid intake. Creating hydration emergency protocols, such as setting minimum water intake goals regardless of schedule changes, helps maintain this crucial aspect of health. Some workers keep electrolyte supplements or beverages on hand specifically for disrupted schedule situations.

Physical activity plans need flexibility during schedule disruptions, but maintaining some form of movement remains important. Having a series of quick, equipment free exercises memorized provides options for maintaining physical activity even when normal workout routines become impossible. These might include basic bodyweight exercises, stretching sequences, or short walking protocols that can be performed almost anywhere, at any time.

Communication protocols form another crucial component of schedule disruption planning. Having predetermined methods for quickly notifying family members, roommates, or other important contacts about sudden schedule changes helps prevent additional stress and confusion. Many workers maintain emergency contact lists and communication templates ready for various disruption scenarios.

Managing light exposure becomes particularly challenging during schedule disruptions, but remains crucial for maintaining circadian rhythm stability as much as possible. Keeping portable light blocking tools like dark glasses or temporary window covering materials accessible helps create sleep promoting environments even in unusual locations or times. Similarly, having access to bright light sources can help promote alertness when needed during unexpected wake periods.

Mental health support strategies become especially important during schedule disruptions. Having predetermined stress management techniques that can be implemented quickly and in various situations helps maintain emotional stability during chaotic periods. This might include breathing exercises, brief meditation protocols, or other calming practices that don't require special equipment or environments.

Recovery planning should be part of any schedule disruption protocol. Understanding how to gradually return to your normal schedule after disruptions helps prevent these temporary changes from becoming longer term problems. This often involves creating a step by step return to normal protocol that can be adjusted based on the duration and severity of the disruption.

Documentation during schedule disruptions helps improve future handling of similar situations. Keeping brief notes about what worked and what didn't during disrupted periods provides valuable information for refining emergency protocols. Many workers maintain simple logs or digital notes specifically for tracking schedule disruptions and their management strategies.

Financial considerations often come into play during schedule disruptions, particularly when they involve additional work hours or unexpected expenses. Having predetermined guidelines for accepting additional shifts or managing overtime helps make quick decisions when needed. Some workers maintain separate emergency funds specifically for managing schedule disruption related expenses.

Support network activation protocols can provide crucial assistance during schedule disruptions. Having predetermined arrangements with family members, friends, or professional services for handling routine responsibilities during emergencies helps prevent these tasks from completely derailing sleep and health routines. This might include childcare backup plans, pet care arrangements, or meal delivery options.

The key to successful schedule disruption management lies in preparation and flexibility. While no emergency plan can account for every possible scenario, having basic protocols in place for sleep, nutrition, activity, and support helps maintain essential wellness practices even when normal routines become impossible. Regular review and updating of these plans ensures they remain relevant and effective as circumstances change.

Holiday Season Survival Guide

The holiday season presents unique challenges for night shift workers who must balance festive obligations with their unconventional schedules. While others enjoy traditional celebrations, those working overnight hours need careful strategies to participate in holiday activities without compromising their health and work performance.

The first key to holiday survival is advance planning. Looking at the holiday calendar months ahead allows you to request strategic time off and arrange schedule adjustments that minimize disruption to your sleep patterns. Many successful night workers choose to concentrate their holiday activities into specific blocks rather than trying to attend every event, helping maintain some schedule consistency during this hectic period.

Managing family expectations becomes crucial during the holiday season. Having honest conversations with loved ones about your schedule limitations helps prevent misunderstandings and resentment. Some night workers find success in creating new traditions that better align with their schedules, such as celebrating Christmas morning on Christmas Eve, or having Thanksgiving dinner at breakfast time.

Sleep management during the holidays requires extra attention. The increased social obligations and daytime events can quickly lead to dangerous levels of sleep debt if not carefully managed. Successful night workers often schedule "recovery days" between major holiday events, using these buffer periods to realign their sleep patterns and prevent exhaustion. Some find it helpful to use vacation days not just for events themselves, but for the day before or after to ensure adequate rest.

Nutrition presents particular challenges during the holiday season. Traditional holiday meals rarely align with optimal eating patterns for night workers, and the abundance of sugary treats can wreak havoc on energy levels during overnight shifts. Creating a holiday nutrition strategy helps maintain stability. This might include eating a protein rich meal before attending holiday gatherings, bringing night shift friendly snacks to events, and being selective about which treats to indulge in based on upcoming work schedules.

The emotional aspects of holiday season survival cannot be overlooked. Many night workers experience increased feelings of isolation during this traditionally social time of year. Building in regular connection points with colleagues who share similar schedules helps combat these feelings. Some workers organize alternative celebrations with their night shift community, creating parallel holiday traditions that honor their unique schedule.

Gift shopping and holiday preparations require different approaches for night workers. While online shopping has made many tasks easier, other holiday activities need creative scheduling. Many night workers use the quiet early morning hours after their shifts for tasks like gift wrapping or holiday decorating, turning potential frustration points into peaceful solo activities.

Managing alcohol consumption becomes particularly important during the holiday season. While others might freely enjoy festive drinks, night workers need to carefully consider how alcohol will affect their sleep patterns and work performance. Many successful night workers develop specific guidelines about which events they'll drink at and which they'll abstain from, based on their work schedule.

Travel planning during the holidays requires extra consideration for night workers. When visiting family or friends in different time zones, the adjustment becomes even more complex than usual. Successful strategies often include arriving a day or two early to adjust, and having clear communications with hosts about sleep scheduling needs.

Maintaining exercise routines through the holiday season helps stabilize energy levels and mood. While traditional gym schedules might not align with holiday obligations, having alternative workout plans ready helps prevent complete disruption of physical activity. Many night workers develop condensed holiday workout routines that can be performed with minimal equipment and time.

Financial planning takes on extra importance during the holiday season, particularly for those earning shift differentials. Many night workers find themselves navigating complex decisions about whether to maintain their premium pay schedules or take time off for holiday events. Creating clear criteria for these decisions in advance helps prevent last minute stress.

Light exposure management becomes particularly challenging during the holiday season, as many celebrations and decorations center around bright lights. Having strategies for managing light exposure, such as wearing blue light blocking glasses during evening family gatherings, helps maintain circadian rhythm stability. Some workers find success in creating specific light exposure protocols for days with holiday events.

The key to holiday season survival lies in selective participation and careful planning. Rather than trying to maintain a normal schedule while adding holiday activities, successful night workers often temporarily adapt their routines to accommodate the season's demands. This might mean choosing specific events to attend while skipping others, or rearranging sleep schedules for important celebrations while maintaining strict sleep discipline on other days.

Recovery planning should be part of any holiday season strategy. Having predetermined protocols for returning to normal routines after holiday disruptions helps prevent seasonal changes from becoming permanent disruptions. This often includes scheduling dedicated recovery periods after major holidays before returning to regular night shift patterns.

The most successful night workers approach the holiday season with a combination of flexibility and boundaries. While willing to adjust their routines for truly important events, they maintain clear limits about which adaptations they'll make and for how long. This balanced approach allows for meaningful participation in holiday traditions while preserving the stability necessary for long term night shift success.

Vacation Planning and Recovery

Planning and taking vacations requires special consideration when you work the night shift. While traditional vacation advice rarely accounts for the unique challenges night workers face, proper planning can make the difference between a truly refreshing break and one that leaves you more exhausted than before.

The first major consideration in vacation planning is the transition period. Unlike day shift workers who can often jump right into vacation mode, night shift workers need to carefully manage their schedule adjustments. Most successful night workers begin gradually shifting their sleep schedule several days before vacation, moving sleep periods by one to two hours each day until they reach a more conventional pattern. This prevents the shock of an abrupt schedule change and allows for better enjoyment of vacation activities.

Choosing the right type of vacation becomes crucial for night shift workers. While all inclusive resorts and guided tours might work well for some, others find that self guided trips offer the flexibility needed to maintain some schedule consistency. Many night workers report success with vacation rentals or private accommodations that allow them to maintain certain aspects of their usual routine while still enjoying new experiences.

The length of vacation also requires careful consideration. While it might seem counterintuitive, longer vacations aren't always better for night shift workers. Many find that trips between five and ten days provide the sweet spot allowing enough time to adjust to a regular schedule and enjoy activities, while not making the return to night shift too difficult. Shorter weekend getaways can be managed without completely disrupting normal sleep patterns, while vacations longer than two weeks often require a more extensive readjustment period upon return.

Recovery time after vacation needs to be built into any travel plans. Successful night workers typically schedule at least two to three days between returning from vacation and resuming work. This buffer period allows for gradual readjustment to night shift patterns and prevents the exhaustion of trying to immediately switch back to overnight hours. Some workers even use this time to maintain a modified schedule, sleeping slightly later each day until they return to their normal pattern.

Time zone considerations add another layer of complexity to vacation planning. While traveling east typically proves easier for night workers since it aligns more naturally with their tendency to be awake at night, westward travel can be more challenging. Many night workers find success in maintaining some aspects of their usual schedule even while traveling, such as staying up later than other travelers or using the early morning hours for activities.

Medication and supplement scheduling during vacation requires advance planning. Those who use sleep aids or supplements to manage their night shift schedule need strategies for adjusting these protocols during vacation. Many work with their healthcare providers to develop specific vacation plans for any sleep or alertness medications, ensuring safe and effective transitions both into and out of vacation mode.

Activity planning takes on special importance during vacations. While day shift workers might naturally gravitate toward traditional touring schedules, night shift workers often find success in alternative timing. Many report enjoying attractions during off peak hours, taking advantage of their comfort with unusual schedules to avoid crowds and experience destinations differently than most tourists.

Nutrition during vacation presents both challenges and opportunities. While completely abandoning night shift eating patterns might seem tempting, maintaining some consistency helps prevent energy crashes and digestive issues. Successful strategies often include keeping some meals at usual times while allowing flexibility for special dining experiences or social occasions.

Managing light exposure during vacation requires conscious effort. While the goal might be to temporarily adapt to a regular schedule, completely abandoning light management can make the return to night shift more difficult. Many workers find success in maintaining some aspects of their usual light exposure patterns, such as avoiding bright light during what would normally be their sleep period, even while enjoying vacation activities.

Exercise and physical activity during vacation need careful consideration. While vacation often means a break from regular workout routines, maintaining some level of physical activity helps prevent complete disruption of circadian rhythms. Many night workers find success in scheduling active pursuits during their usual wake hours, even while on vacation.

Family and social dynamics during vacation require clear communication. When traveling with others who don't work night shift, setting expectations about schedule needs and energy patterns helps prevent misunderstandings. Some workers find success in taking solo time during hours when they would normally be awake, allowing for both social activities and personal space.

Financial planning for vacations takes on additional complexity for night shift workers. Beyond standard vacation costs, considerations might include premium pay lost during time off, additional recovery days needed, and the potential need for private accommodations to maintain sleep quality. Many successful night workers build these factors into their vacation budgets and planning.

The return to work phase after vacation requires as much planning as the vacation itself. Having a detailed protocol for returning to night shift helps prevent the post vacation blues from becoming a major disruption. This often includes specific sleep scheduling, light exposure patterns, and nutrition plans for the days leading up to return to work.

The most successful night shift vacations balance the desire for traditional experiences with the realities of an adapted circadian rhythm. While some schedule disruption proves inevitable, thoughtful planning can minimize its impact and allow for truly restful and enjoyable breaks from routine. The key lies in accepting that night shift vacations might look different from conventional ones, while still providing all the benefits of time away from work.

Managing Doctor Appointments and Daytime Obligations

Managing daytime appointments and obligations presents unique challenges for night shift workers who need to navigate a world that operates on a traditional schedule. While most businesses, medical offices, and service providers maintain standard business hours, night workers can develop effective strategies to meet these obligations without sacrificing their health and rest.

The most crucial aspect of managing daytime appointments involves strategic scheduling. Whenever possible, aim to schedule appointments for late afternoon, typically around 3 or 4 PM. This timing allows for adequate sleep after a night shift while still meeting obligations before the next shift begins. Many medical offices and service providers now offer extended hours, and specifically requesting these later appointments can make a significant difference in maintaining schedule stability.

When early appointments prove unavoidable, careful sleep management becomes essential. Rather than attempting to maintain normal sleep patterns, successful night workers often opt for a split sleep schedule on appointment days. This might involve sleeping for 4-5 hours immediately after work, attending the appointment, then getting another 2-3 hours of sleep before the next shift. While not ideal for regular use, this approach helps manage occasional daytime obligations without creating severe sleep debt.

Communication with healthcare providers and service professionals about night shift status often yields unexpected accommodations. Many providers, once aware of the situation, willingly offer flexibility in scheduling or suggest alternative solutions. Some medical practices even maintain specific appointment slots for night shift workers, recognizing the growing number of patients working unconventional hours.

Banking, legal matters, and other professional services require similar strategic planning. Online and mobile services have greatly expanded access for night workers, but some matters still demand in person attention. Many night workers successfully batch these obligations, scheduling multiple appointments for the same day to minimize sleep disruption. This approach might mean more tiredness on a single day but prevents multiple schedule disruptions throughout the month.

Child related obligations present particular challenges for night shift working parents. School meetings, sports events, and medical appointments often occur during traditional daytime hours. Successful night shift parents often coordinate with partners or family members to share these responsibilities, but when personal attendance proves necessary, they develop specific recovery plans for these days. This might include abbreviated workout routines, modified nutrition protocols, and adjusted sleep schedules.

Vehicle maintenance, home repairs, and similar services typically operate during daylight hours. Many night workers find success in developing relationships with service providers who understand their schedule constraints. Some auto repair shops, for instance, offer early drop off options with secure key drops, allowing night workers to leave vehicles before heading home to sleep. Similarly, some home service providers will work with night shift clients to schedule appointments at the beginning or end of their business day.

Government and administrative obligations often prove less flexible than private services. For tasks like driver's license renewal, jury duty, or court appearances, night workers must carefully plan around mandated times. Successful strategies include using vacation days strategically, arranging shift swaps with colleagues, and when possible, requesting schedule accommodations through proper channels. Some jurisdictions now offer expanded hours for certain services, recognizing the needs of night shift workers.

Regular personal care appointments such as dental visits, haircuts, or medical check ups can be scheduled with more flexibility. Many night workers establish relationships with providers who maintain early or late hours, allowing for appointments that align better with their schedule. Some even find providers who specifically cater to night shift workers, offering hours and services designed around unconventional schedules.

Emergency situations require special consideration and advance planning. Having a clear protocol for handling unexpected daytime obligations helps prevent panic and excessive stress. This might include maintaining a list of colleagues willing to provide shift coverage, having pre arranged child care options, and keeping an emergency fund for unexpected schedule adjustments. Many successful night workers also maintain relationships with 24 hour service providers for situations that cannot wait for traditional business hours.

Documentation and record keeping become particularly important when managing daytime obligations. Keeping detailed records of appointments, including travel time, actual appointment duration, and recovery periods helps in planning future obligations more effectively. Many night workers maintain separate calendars for day obligations, allowing them to visualize and manage schedule impacts more effectively.

Technology can significantly ease the burden of managing daytime obligations. Calendar apps with multiple time zone capabilities help track appointments in relation to sleep schedules. Reminder systems adjusted for night shift timing prevent missed obligations. Additionally, many services now offer online scheduling, virtual appointments, and automated systems that work around the clock, providing alternatives to traditional daytime appointments.

The most successful night shift workers approach daytime obligations as a manageable challenge rather than an insurmountable obstacle. While the traditional business world may not fully accommodate night shift schedules, creative planning, clear communication, and strategic use of available resources can help maintain both professional obligations and personal well being. The key lies in developing systems that work within individual constraints while minimizing disruption to established routines.

The Night Shift Home Office

Creating an effective home office setup for night shift work requires careful consideration of both environmental and practical factors. While many night workers focus primarily on their workplace environment, having a properly equipped home office space can significantly enhance productivity during nontraditional hours and provide a dedicated area for handling personal business matters.

The foundation of any night shift home office begins with appropriate lighting. Unlike traditional home offices that benefit from natural light, night workers need to create an environment that maintains alertness without disrupting their circadian rhythms. Full spectrum LED lighting with adjustable brightness and color temperature proves invaluable. During active work hours, cooler, brighter lights help maintain alertness, while warmer, dimmer settings can be used during wind down periods. Installing smart lighting systems allows for automated adjustments that match your specific schedule.

Sound management takes on special importance in a night shift home office. While the world sleeps, ambient noise levels drop significantly, making even minor sounds more noticeable and potentially distracting. Consider installing sound dampening panels or using white noise machines to create a consistent acoustic environment. Quality noise canceling headphones can prove essential for focused work, especially if other household members are active during your work hours.

Temperature control plays a crucial role in maintaining comfort and alertness during overnight hours. Our body temperature naturally drops during nighttime, which can lead to drowsiness. Maintaining a slightly cooler room temperature, typically between 65 and 68 degrees Fahrenheit, helps combat this natural tendency. A dedicated thermostat or space heater with timer functions allows for automated temperature adjustments that align with your schedule.

Ergonomics become even more critical during night hours when our bodies are naturally more susceptible to fatigue and discomfort. Invest in a high quality adjustable chair that provides proper lumbar support and promotes good posture. An adjustable height desk, whether standing or sitting, allows for position changes that help maintain alertness and reduce physical strain. Proper monitor positioning, ergonomic keyboards, and appropriate mouse support complete the foundation of a comfortable workspace.

Organization takes on additional importance in a night shift home office. When operating during unconventional hours, quick access to essential items and information becomes crucial. Develop a filing system that accommodates both physical and digital documents, ensuring easy retrieval during times when outside assistance may be unavailable. Label makers, color coding systems, and digital organization tools help maintain order and efficiency.

Technology selection requires careful consideration of night shift specific needs. Choose computers and monitors with blue light filtering capabilities and night modes. Install software that automatically adjusts screen temperature based on time of day. Ensure all equipment operates quietly to minimize disturbance during sensitive hours. Having reliable backup systems becomes especially important when technical support may be unavailable during your active hours.

Communication tools require particular attention in a night shift home office. While email remains accessible around the clock, other communication methods may need adaptation. Consider installing a dedicated phone line with customizable quiet hours for voicemail. Video conferencing setups should include appropriate lighting for clear visibility during virtual meetings that may occur during your active hours but others' sleep time.

Storage solutions in a night shift home office should prioritize accessibility while maintaining organization. Consider installing cabinet systems with soft close features to minimize noise. Use clear storage containers to easily identify contents without opening containers. Implement a system for temporary storage of items that require daytime attention, ensuring nothing gets overlooked during schedule transitions.

Privacy considerations take on added importance when working unconventional hours. Window treatments should provide complete light control while maintaining security. Position computer screens to prevent visibility from outside, particularly during dark hours when indoor lighting makes displays more visible through windows. Consider installing privacy film on windows to maintain natural light access during daytime sleep hours while ensuring security.

Maintenance of a night shift home office requires different protocols than traditional spaces. Develop cleaning routines that align with your schedule without creating noise that might disturb others. Keep basic repair tools and supplies readily available for addressing minor issues during hours when maintenance services are unavailable. Establish regular equipment check schedules to prevent failures during critical periods.

Emergency preparedness becomes particularly important in a night shift home office. Install battery backup systems for essential equipment to handle power interruptions during overnight hours. Keep emergency lighting easily accessible. Maintain a list of 24 hour service providers for critical systems. Consider installing a small refrigerator and microwave to maintain access to nutrition during hours when kitchen access might disturb others.

The psychological aspects of a night shift home office deserve careful consideration. Personalize the space with elements that promote alertness and positivity during night hours. Consider incorporating plants that thrive in artificial light. Display motivational elements that reinforce the benefits of your chosen schedule. Create distinct zones for different activities to help maintain work life boundaries despite unconventional hours.

Success in maintaining a night shift home office ultimately depends on regular evaluation and adjustment of the space to meet evolving needs. Schedule periodic reviews of office functionality, considering changes in work requirements and personal preferences. Remain open to incorporating new technologies and organizational systems that might better serve your unique schedule demands.

Financial Planning for Night Premium Pay

Financial planning takes on unique dimensions for those working night shifts, particularly due to the premium pay that often accompanies these unconventional hours. While the additional compensation can provide significant financial advantages, it requires careful management to maximize its benefits and create long term stability.

Night shift differential pay typically ranges from 5% to 15% above base salary, though some industries offer even higher premiums during certain hours or holidays. This additional income presents both opportunities and potential pitfalls. The key is developing a strategic approach that accounts for both the immediate benefits and long term implications of this compensation structure.

One critical aspect of night shift financial planning involves understanding the true value of your premium pay. Beyond the basic percentage increase, consider how this additional income affects your tax bracket, benefit calculations, and overall compensation package. Many night workers make the mistake of viewing premium pay as purely disposable income, rather than incorporating it into their comprehensive financial strategy.

Creating a sustainable budget that accounts for the irregular nature of night shift premiums proves essential. Some organizations adjust premium rates based on specific hours or seasonal needs, while others might modify shift differential policies over time. Building your core budget around your base pay while developing specific allocations for premium income helps maintain financial stability regardless of scheduling changes.

Investment strategies should reflect the unique earning patterns of night shift work. Consider establishing automatic investment transfers that coincide with premium pay deposits, taking advantage of dollar cost averaging while ensuring this additional income contributes to long term wealth building. Many successful night workers designate specific percentages of their premium pay for retirement accounts, emergency funds, and other investment vehicles.

Emergency fund planning takes on special importance for night shift workers. The physical and mental demands of overnight work can sometimes necessitate unexpected breaks or schedule changes. Maintaining a robust emergency fund, ideally containing six to twelve months of expenses, provides crucial flexibility when adapting to the challenges of night shift work. Consider allocating a portion of your premium pay specifically to building and maintaining this safety net.

Insurance considerations deserve careful attention when working nights. Review how your premium pay affects life insurance calculations and disability coverage. Some policies offer special provisions for shift workers, while others might have exclusions or limitations related to overnight work. Understanding these nuances helps ensure adequate protection for you and your dependents.

Retirement planning should account for both the advantages and potential challenges of night shift work. While higher earnings can enable increased retirement contributions, the physical demands of night work might influence your desired retirement timeline. Consider working with financial advisors who understand the specific needs of night shift workers and can help develop retirement strategies that align with your unique circumstances.

Tax planning becomes more complex with night shift premium pay. Consult with tax professionals who can help optimize your withholdings and identify deductions specific to night workers. Some expenses related to maintaining a night shift schedule, such as blackout curtains or specialized sleep equipment, might qualify for tax benefits under certain circumstances.

Real estate and mortgage planning should factor in the stability of your premium pay. While lenders often consider shift differentials when calculating borrowing capacity, they may require longer work history to verify the consistency of this income. Developing a clear documentation system for your premium earnings helps strengthen your position when seeking mortgage approval or refinancing options.

Debt management strategies should prioritize the strategic use of premium pay. Consider accelerating debt repayment using shift differentials while maintaining base salary for regular expenses. This approach can significantly reduce interest costs over time while preserving financial flexibility. Many successful night workers designate specific premium shifts for debt reduction, creating clear goals and measurable progress.

Education and skill development investments deserve consideration in your financial planning. Some organizations offer additional premium pay for specialized certifications or advanced training. Allocating a portion of your current premium pay toward education expenses can lead to increased earning potential and career advancement opportunities.

Family financial planning requires special attention when premium pay constitutes a significant portion of household income. Develop clear communication systems with family members about financial goals and spending priorities. Consider establishing separate accounts for premium pay to facilitate better tracking and allocation of these funds.

Long term care and disability planning become particularly important given the physical demands of night shift work. Research suggests that long term night shift work may increase certain health risks, making insurance coverage and healthcare savings essential components of your financial strategy. Consider allocating a portion of premium pay specifically for health related savings accounts or insurance premiums.

Success in managing night shift premium pay ultimately depends on developing and maintaining clear financial systems that account for both the opportunities and challenges of unconventional work hours.

Regular review and adjustment of your financial strategy ensures continued alignment with your goals while maximizing the benefits of your premium compensation.

Career Development on Night Shift

C areer development presents unique challenges and opportunities for night shift workers. While many advancement opportunities traditionally occur during daylight hours, strategic professionals can leverage the distinctive aspects of overnight work to accelerate their career growth and create compelling advancement paths.

The fundamental key to career development on night shift lies in visibility management. Since many organizational leaders and decision makers work during traditional hours, night workers must be intentional about creating awareness of their contributions and capabilities. This often requires developing strong documentation practices, maintaining detailed shift reports, and finding creative ways to showcase achievements that occur while others sleep.

Leadership opportunities often emerge more readily during night shifts, particularly in industries with reduced overnight staffing. Taking initiative during critical situations, managing emergency responses, and demonstrating independent decision making abilities can rapidly build a reputation for reliability and competence. Many successful night shift workers have accelerated their career progression by embracing these autonomous roles and documenting their impact.

Mentorship dynamics shift dramatically during overnight hours. While traditional mentoring relationships might prove challenging to maintain, night workers often develop powerful peer mentoring networks. These relationships can provide crucial guidance, support, and professional development opportunities. Additionally, serving as a mentor to newer night shift workers demonstrates leadership capability and strengthens organizational value.

Professional development activities require careful planning when working nights. Many training programs, seminars, and networking events occur during traditional business hours. Successful night shift professionals often negotiate flexible training schedules, utilize online learning platforms, and create customized development plans that accommodate their unique schedules. Some organizations offer specialized training sessions for night staff, presenting opportunities for both skill development and increased visibility.

Building relationships with daytime colleagues demands intentional effort. Scheduling occasional overlap meetings, participating in cross shift projects, and maintaining active communication through digital platforms helps bridge the temporal divide. Many night shift workers find success by arriving early to attend key meetings or staying late to connect with daytime leadership, strategically managing these interactions to maximize their impact while maintaining work life balance.

Industry specific certifications and advanced training often enhance career prospects for night workers. Many facilities offer additional compensation or advancement opportunities for specialized skills particularly valuable during overnight hours. Identifying and pursuing these certifications can create clear advancement paths while increasing immediate earning potential.

Project management opportunities frequently emerge during night shifts, particularly for infrastructure updates, system maintenance, or process improvements that prove disruptive during peak hours. Taking ownership of these initiatives provides valuable experience while demonstrating capability to upper management. Successful night shift professionals often actively seek out these projects, viewing them as stepping stones to broader responsibilities.

Remote work and global team opportunities have expanded significantly for night shift workers, particularly in industries operating across multiple time zones. Many organizations value team members comfortable with overnight schedules for international collaboration. Building expertise in virtual team management and cross cultural communication can open new career paths previously unavailable to night workers.

Documentation and process improvement initiatives present significant career development opportunities during overnight hours. Many organizations struggle with standardizing procedures across shifts. Night workers who take initiative in developing and implementing improved protocols often gain recognition as valuable organizational assets. This operational expertise can lead to advancement into process improvement or quality management roles.

Networking strategies require adaptation for night shift professionals. While traditional networking events might prove challenging to attend, industry specific online communities, professional social media platforms, and virtual conferences offer alternative connection opportunities. Many successful night shift workers build robust professional networks by engaging with international colleagues working similar hours.

Educational advancement often aligns well with night shift schedules, particularly through online learning platforms and flexible degree programs. Many night workers successfully pursue advanced degrees or professional certifications during their off hours, leveraging the quieter daytime period for focused study. This academic progression, combined with practical overnight experience, creates compelling qualifications for advancement.

Leadership development takes on unique dimensions during night shifts. The autonomous nature of overnight work often requires developing strong decision making capabilities, crisis management skills, and team coordination abilities. Documenting these experiences and translating them into demonstrated leadership competencies proves crucial for career advancement discussions.

Cross training initiatives present valuable development opportunities during overnight hours. Reduced staffing often requires night workers to develop broader skill sets than their daytime counterparts. Actively pursuing cross training opportunities not only increases immediate value to the organization but also creates flexibility for future career moves.

Success in night shift career development ultimately depends on proactive management of both opportunities and challenges. Creating visibility for overnight achievements, maintaining strong professional networks despite unconventional hours, and continuously developing relevant skills enables career growth even within the constraints of night shift schedules. The key lies in viewing the unique aspects of overnight work not as limitations but as distinctive advantages in professional development.

Building Professional Relationships

Building professional relationships presents unique challenges and opportunities for night shift workers. The unconventional schedule can make traditional networking and relationship building seem daunting, but with intentional strategies and consistent effort, night workers can develop robust professional networks that support their career growth and job satisfaction.

The foundation of professional relationships on night shift begins with your immediate team. The shared experience of working unconventional hours often creates strong bonds between night shift colleagues. These relationships tend to develop more depth than typical workplace connections, as night teams frequently face challenging situations together with limited outside support. Nurturing these connections through active listening, reliable support, and genuine interest in colleagues' lives creates a strong professional foundation.

Cross shift relationships require particular attention and strategy. While you might rarely see your daytime counterparts in person, maintaining strong connections across shifts proves crucial for operational continuity and career development. Successful night workers often schedule brief overlap periods to connect with incoming or outgoing shifts, using this time to share critical information and build rapport. Digital communication tools, shared documentation systems, and occasional scheduled meetups help bridge the temporal divide.

Leadership relationships demand creative approaches when working nights. Since most organizational leaders work traditional hours, night shift workers must actively create opportunities for interaction and visibility. This might involve occasionally adjusting your schedule to attend important meetings, providing detailed reports that highlight your contributions, or scheduling regular check ins during overlap periods. Many successful night workers find that arriving early or staying late once or twice a month for face to face meetings with leadership pays significant dividends in professional relationship development.

Mentorship takes on different dimensions during night shifts. While traditional mentoring relationships might prove challenging to maintain, night workers often develop valuable peer mentoring networks. These relationships provide crucial support, knowledge sharing, and professional guidance. Additionally, serving as a mentor to newer night shift workers not only helps others succeed but also strengthens your own professional network and leadership capabilities.

Industry connections beyond your immediate workplace require strategic cultivation when working nights. Professional associations, online communities, and social media platforms provide valuable networking opportunities that align with night shift schedules. Many successful night workers build connections with international colleagues working similar hours, creating global professional networks that enhance their career prospects and knowledge base.

Vendor and supplier relationships often become particularly important during night shifts, as these connections can prove crucial when facing operational challenges with limited immediate support. Building strong relationships with key service providers, maintaining updated contact information, and understanding escalation protocols helps ensure successful problem resolution during overnight hours. These relationships frequently develop into valuable professional connections that extend beyond immediate operational needs.

Interdepartmental relationships require special attention during night shifts. While different departments might operate with minimal overlap during overnight hours, maintaining strong connections across functional areas helps ensure operational success and creates opportunities for professional growth. Regular communication, shared project work, and mutual support during challenging situations strengthen these vital organizational relationships.

Professional relationships with industry peers working similar schedules provide valuable support networks and learning opportunities. Many night workers find success in creating informal professional groups that meet during hours convenient for overnight schedules. These connections offer opportunities to share best practices, discuss common challenges, and develop innovative solutions to night shift specific issues.

Remote team relationships have become increasingly important as organizations expand their global operations. Night shift workers often find themselves collaborating with international colleagues, requiring skills in virtual relationship building and cross cultural communication. Developing expertise in maintaining strong professional connections across time zones and cultures creates valuable capabilities for career advancement.

Educational and training relationships benefit from intentional cultivation during night shifts. Connecting with instructors, academic advisors, and fellow students might require additional planning, but these relationships prove valuable for professional development. Many successful night workers maintain strong connections with educational institutions and training providers, creating opportunities for continuous learning and skill development.

Community relationships take on special significance for night shift workers, as these connections help combat the isolation that can accompany unconventional schedules. Engaging with community organizations, professional groups, and volunteer opportunities during compatible hours helps build a broader professional network while contributing to personal fulfillment and work life balance.

The success of professional relationships during night shifts ultimately depends on consistent effort, creative scheduling, and genuine engagement. While the unconventional hours present unique challenges, they also create distinctive opportunities for building strong professional networks. The key lies in viewing these relationships as essential investments in both current job success and long term career development.

Regular maintenance of professional relationships requires dedicated attention during night shifts. Setting reminders for check ins, scheduling periodic face to face meetings, and actively participating in digital professional communities helps ensure these vital connections remain strong despite unconventional hours. Many successful night workers maintain relationship development calendars, ensuring no important professional connection gets neglected due to schedule challenges.

Building and maintaining professional relationships during night shifts ultimately requires a combination of intentional strategy and genuine engagement. While the unconventional schedule presents unique challenges, it also offers opportunities to develop distinctive professional networks that span traditional time boundaries. Success comes from viewing these relationship building efforts not as additional tasks but as essential components of professional growth and job satisfaction.

Personal Development During Down Hours

The overnight hours offer unique opportunities for personal development that day shift workers often struggle to find. While others sleep, night shift workers can leverage quiet periods for self improvement and growth. The key lies in strategic planning and consistent execution of personal development activities that align with the natural rhythms of overnight work.

Reading and learning tend to peak during the middle hours of night shift, when mental alertness remains high but operational demands often decrease. Many successful night workers develop extensive knowledge bases by dedicating specific hours to focused study. Whether pursuing formal education, professional certifications, or personal interests, the relative quiet of night shift provides an ideal environment for deep learning and reflection.

Online courses and digital learning platforms have revolutionized personal development opportunities for night shift workers. The ability to access high quality educational content at any hour allows for consistent skill development without schedule conflicts. Many night workers find success in breaking larger courses into manageable segments that fit naturally into their work patterns, completing modules during slower periods and reviewing materials during high energy hours.

Creative pursuits flourish during night shifts, as the peaceful atmosphere often enhances focus and imagination. Writers, artists, and musicians working nights frequently report increased productivity during overnight hours. The reduced external stimulation and limited interruptions create ideal conditions for creative development, whether working on personal projects or developing new professional skills.

Language learning represents another area where night shift workers often excel. The quiet hours provide perfect conditions for pronunciation practice, while international connections across time zones offer opportunities for real time language exchange. Many successful night workers develop multilingual capabilities by combining structured learning during work hours with practical application through global professional networks.

Financial education and personal business development benefit from the focused attention possible during night shifts. Many workers use this time to study investment strategies, develop side businesses, or enhance their understanding of personal finance. The ability to concentrate on complex financial concepts without daily distractions accelerates learning and implementation of wealth building strategies.

Technical skills development aligns naturally with night shift schedules. Whether learning programming languages, mastering new software platforms, or developing technical certifications, the uninterrupted time allows for deep focus on complex technical concepts. Many night workers significantly advance their technical capabilities by dedicating specific hours to hands on practice and study.

Personal wellness education takes on special significance during night shifts. Understanding the unique health challenges of overnight work leads many to develop expertise in sleep science, nutrition, and stress management. This knowledge not only benefits personal health but often transforms night workers into valuable resources for colleagues facing similar challenges.

Leadership development during night shifts often follows unconventional paths. While traditional leadership programs might prove challenging to attend, many night workers develop strong leadership capabilities through practical experience, online learning, and mentoring relationships. The autonomous nature of night work frequently provides opportunities to demonstrate and develop leadership skills in real world situations.

Writing and communication skills often improve significantly during night shifts. Many workers use the quiet hours to develop blogs, write articles, or create content related to their professional expertise. This practice not only enhances communication abilities but often leads to recognition as thought leaders in their fields.

Project management skills naturally develop during night shifts, as workers frequently need to manage complex tasks with limited immediate support. Many successful night workers leverage this experience by pursuing formal project management education during quiet hours, combining practical experience with theoretical knowledge.

Personal organization and productivity systems benefit from the focused attention possible during night shifts. Many workers use this time to develop and refine their organizational systems, creating efficient workflows that enhance both professional performance and personal life management.

The development of emotional intelligence and interpersonal skills might seem challenging during night shifts, but many workers find success through focused study and practical application. Understanding personality types, communication styles, and conflict resolution techniques during quiet hours prepares workers for effective interaction during busier periods.

Time management mastery often emerges as a crucial personal development area for night shift workers. The unique challenges of balancing work, sleep, and personal life lead many to develop sophisticated time management systems. This expertise frequently transfers to other areas of life and career advancement.

Meditation and mindfulness practices find natural homes during night shifts. Many workers use quiet periods for developing these skills, leading to improved stress management and enhanced personal awareness. The peaceful overnight environment often proves ideal for establishing and maintaining contemplative practices.

The key to successful personal development during night shifts lies in creating sustainable systems that align with natural energy patterns and work demands. Understanding personal peak performance times, identifying available learning windows, and maintaining consistent development habits ensures steady progress despite unconventional schedules.

Long-Term Health Considerations

Working the night shift presents unique long term health considerations that require careful attention and proactive management. While the human body can adapt remarkably well to overnight work, sustained exposure to circadian disruption necessitates specific strategies to protect and maintain health over years or decades of night shift work.

Cardiovascular health emerges as a primary concern for career night workers. The disruption of normal sleep wake cycles can impact blood pressure regulation and heart rhythms. Research indicates higher rates of cardiovascular disease among long term night workers, making preventive measures essential. Regular cardiovascular screening, consistent exercise routines, and careful attention to diet become crucial tools for protecting heart health.

Metabolic impacts of sustained night work deserve special consideration. The body's natural glucose regulation and hormone production follow circadian patterns that night work disrupts. Long term night workers often face increased risks of diabetes and metabolic disorders. Managing these risks requires careful attention to meal timing, regular blood sugar monitoring, and lifestyle choices that support metabolic health.

Bone density presents another area requiring proactive management. Reduced exposure to natural sunlight can impact vitamin D production, potentially leading to decreased bone density over time. Successful career night workers often combine careful supplementation with strategic sunlight exposure and weight bearing exercise to maintain bone health.

Immune system function requires special attention during extended periods of night work. The complex relationship between sleep, circadian rhythms, and immune response means night workers must take extra precautions to support their immune systems. Regular health screenings, appropriate vaccination schedules, and immune supporting lifestyle choices become essential.

Cognitive health represents a crucial consideration for long term night workers. While the brain demonstrates remarkable adaptability, sustained circadian disruption may impact memory, learning, and cognitive processing over time. Successful career night workers often incorporate specific cognitive training exercises and lifestyle choices that support brain health.

Digestive health frequently emerges as a challenge during extended night work. The misalignment between eating patterns and natural digestive rhythms can lead to various gastrointestinal issues. Managing these challenges requires careful attention to eating patterns, food choices, and digestive support strategies that align with overnight schedules.

Hormonal balance presents unique challenges for long term night workers. The complex interplay between circadian rhythms and hormone production means night workers must pay special attention to endocrine health. Regular hormone level monitoring and lifestyle choices that support hormonal balance become increasingly important over time.

Cancer risk factors associated with long term night work require serious consideration. Research suggests potential links between sustained circadian disruption and certain cancer types. While causation remains under study, successful career night workers often incorporate additional cancer screening protocols and preventive measures into their health routines.

Mental health impacts of sustained night work demand ongoing attention. While many workers successfully adapt to overnight schedules, long term exposure to circadian disruption can influence mood regulation and emotional well being. Maintaining robust mental health support systems and regular psychological check ins becomes crucial for career sustainability.

Vision health requires specific consideration for night workers. Extended exposure to artificial light, particularly during natural darkness hours, may impact eye health over time. Regular vision screening, appropriate light exposure management, and eye health protocols become essential for long term night workers.

Reproductive health considerations vary by gender but remain important for all night workers. The impact of circadian disruption on reproductive hormones and fertility requires attention, particularly for workers planning families. Understanding these impacts and working with healthcare providers to monitor reproductive health becomes crucial.

Musculoskeletal health often faces unique challenges during night work. The combination of irregular sleep patterns and physical demands can impact posture, muscle tension, and joint health. Successful career night workers typically incorporate specific physical therapy protocols and ergonomic considerations into their routines.

Aging presents distinct considerations for night shift workers. As the body's natural ability to adapt to circadian disruption changes with age, many workers find they need to adjust their health management strategies over time. Understanding these changes and developing appropriate adaptation strategies becomes crucial for career longevity.

The key to managing long term health while working nights lies in developing comprehensive, sustainable health monitoring and maintenance systems. Regular health screenings, proactive lifestyle choices, and careful attention to emerging research on shift work health impacts allow many workers to maintain successful careers on overnight schedules. Understanding personal risk factors, maintaining open communication with healthcare providers, and adjusting health management strategies as needed ensures the best possible outcomes for career night workers.

When to Consider a Schedule Change

The decision to transition away from night shift work represents one of the most significant choices a career night worker can face. While many professionals successfully maintain overnight schedules for decades, there comes a time when some workers need to seriously evaluate whether continuing night work serves their best interests. This evaluation requires careful consideration of multiple factors and honest self assessment.

Physical health often serves as a primary indicator when considering a schedule change. As we age, our bodies may become less adaptable to circadian disruption. Some workers find that despite following all the recommended protocols for night shift success, they begin experiencing persistent health issues that don't resolve with standard interventions. These might include chronic sleep problems, digestive issues that resist dietary changes, or cardiovascular concerns that become harder to manage on a night schedule.

Family dynamics frequently drive schedule change considerations. While many night workers successfully balance family life with overnight work, major life changes can alter this equation. The arrival of children, aging parents requiring care, or changes in a partner's schedule might necessitate reevaluating work hours. Sometimes, the emotional toll of missing family events or struggling to maintain meaningful connections pushes workers to consider transitioning to traditional hours.

Career advancement opportunities sometimes influence schedule decisions. While many organizations value and promote night workers, some career paths may require a move to daytime hours. Workers must weigh the benefits of night shift premiums against potential career growth opportunities available during traditional business hours. This calculation varies significantly by industry and individual circumstance.

Social isolation can become increasingly challenging over time. Even with strong support networks and careful attention to maintaining relationships, some workers find that the cumulative effect of living on an opposite schedule from most of society becomes emotionally draining. When social connections consistently suffer despite best efforts to maintain them, it may signal time to consider a schedule change.

Quality of life assessments play a crucial role in schedule change decisions. Workers should regularly evaluate how well their current schedule aligns with their life goals and values. This includes considering factors like personal hobbies, educational pursuits, community involvement, and overall life satisfaction. When night work consistently interferes with achieving important life goals, schedule changes merit serious consideration.

Financial considerations often impact timing of schedule changes. Night shift premiums can represent significant income, making transitions to day shifts financially challenging. Workers considering schedule changes need to carefully evaluate their financial situation, including potential impacts on benefits, retirement planning, and overall household budget. Sometimes, strategic financial planning can make schedule transitions more feasible.

Age related factors deserve special attention when considering schedule changes. Research suggests that older workers often find night shifts increasingly challenging to maintain. Changes in sleep patterns, reduced physical resilience, and altered circadian adaptability can make overnight work more difficult with age. Understanding these natural changes helps workers make informed decisions about schedule transitions.

Workplace environment changes sometimes necessitate schedule reevaluation. Organizations may alter shift structures, change staffing models, or modify work expectations in ways that impact the viability of night work. When workplace changes significantly affect job satisfaction or work life balance, workers may need to consider schedule alternatives.

Health care provider recommendations occasionally drive schedule change decisions. Medical professionals familiar with a worker's specific health situation may advise transitioning away from night work. While such recommendations should be carefully evaluated in context, they often provide valuable insight into potential health impacts of continued night work.

Personal readiness for change requires honest assessment. Successfully transitioning from night work often depends on proper preparation and timing. Workers should evaluate their readiness for major lifestyle changes, including impacts on daily routines, relationships, and personal habits. Sometimes, delaying schedule changes until better prepared improves transition success.

Support system availability influences transition timing. Strong support networks can make schedule changes more manageable. Workers should assess whether they have necessary emotional, practical, and professional support to successfully navigate schedule transitions. Building these support systems before initiating changes often improves outcomes.

Alternative schedule options deserve thorough exploration. Before completely abandoning night work, some workers benefit from considering intermediate solutions like rotating shifts, partial schedule changes, or alternative work arrangements. Understanding all available options helps workers make informed decisions about schedule changes.

The decision to change schedules requires careful planning and preparation. Those choosing to transition away from night work benefit from developing comprehensive transition plans that address financial, professional, personal, and health considerations. Successful transitions often involve gradual changes and careful attention to maintaining stability during the adjustment period.

Creating Your Sustainable Night Shift Lifestyle

Creating a sustainable night shift lifestyle represents the culmination of all the strategies, habits, and practices covered throughout this book. The key to long term success lies not in perfectly executing every recommendation, but in developing a personalized approach that works for your unique situation and can be maintained consistently over time.

Sustainability starts with accepting that your lifestyle will look different from the conventional daytime worker. Rather than constantly fighting against your schedule or viewing it as temporary, embrace the distinct rhythm of night work. This mental shift allows you to fully invest in creating routines and systems that support your wellbeing rather than just surviving until you can return to "normal" hours.

The foundation of a sustainable night shift lifestyle rests on sleep consistency. While perfect sleep may not be achievable every day, establishing and protecting your primary sleep schedule most days creates stability. This means maintaining similar sleep and wake times even on days off whenever possible. Occasional deviations for special events or obligations become manageable when they're exceptions rather than the rule.

Nutritional sustainability requires developing practical eating patterns that can be maintained long term. This means finding a balance between optimal nutrition timing and real world constraints. Rather than attempting to follow overly rigid meal schedules, focus on consistent eating windows that work with your specific job duties and lifestyle. Stock your home and workplace with healthy options that are readily available during your active hours.

Physical activity needs to fit naturally into your schedule rather than feeling like another obligation. Identify exercise times that consistently work with your energy levels and commitments. This might mean shorter, more frequent movement sessions rather than traditional lengthy workouts. The key is establishing patterns you can maintain week after week without exhausting yourself or creating schedule stress.

Social connections require ongoing cultivation but shouldn't create constant strain. Build your social circle to include other night workers when possible. Develop communication routines with family and friends that work within your schedule constraints. Use technology thoughtfully to maintain relationships during opposite hours. Accept that some events will be missed while prioritizing the connections most important to you.

Career development on night shift becomes sustainable when you take a long view approach. Rather than trying to participate in every daytime opportunity, focus on building skills and relationships that align with your schedule. Look for mentors who understand night work and can help guide your growth. Document your contributions and achievements so they're visible to decision makers who may not directly observe your work.

Financial stability plays a crucial role in sustainability. Build your budget around your base pay rather than relying heavily on shift differentials or overtime. This creates flexibility to adjust hours if needed while maintaining financial security. Consider how your schedule affects expenses like childcare, meal costs, and transportation when planning your long term financial strategy.

Mental health sustainability requires proactive maintenance rather than crisis management. Develop regular check in routines to monitor your psychological wellbeing. Build a support network that includes both professional resources and personal connections who understand night work challenges. Create decompression rituals that help you process stress and maintain emotional balance.

Home environment optimization becomes increasingly important for long term success. Invest in quality light blocking solutions, temperature control, and sound management for your sleeping space. Create designated areas for daytime relaxation that don't interfere with sleep zones. Make your living space work for your schedule rather than constantly adapting to conventional layouts and routines.

Family dynamics require ongoing attention and adjustment as circumstances change. Establish clear communication protocols about schedule needs while remaining flexible when possible. Create special traditions and connection points that work within your timing constraints. Help family members understand and respect your schedule requirements while finding creative ways to maintain meaningful involvement in their lives.

Professional boundaries become essential for sustainability. Learn to effectively communicate your schedule limitations to colleagues and supervisors. Develop systems for handling daytime meetings and responsibilities that don't consistently disrupt your sleep. Build professional relationships that respect your time constraints while allowing you to fully contribute to your organization.

Personal development needs to align with your natural energy patterns and available time. Choose growth opportunities that complement rather than conflict with your schedule. This might mean selecting online learning options, finding night shift study groups, or creating independent project timelines that work within your hours.

The most sustainable night shift lifestyle emerges from consistent small choices rather than dramatic changes. Focus on gradual improvements in each area of wellbeing. Celebrate progress while accepting that some days will flow better than others. Remember that sustainability means finding balance between ideal practices and practical realities.

Long term success on night shift requires regular reassessment and adjustment of your systems. Schedule periodic reviews of how well your routines are working. Be willing to modify approaches that no longer serve your needs while maintaining core practices that support your wellbeing. Think of sustainability as an ongoing process rather than a fixed destination.

Your sustainable night shift lifestyle will likely look different from others, even those working similar schedules. The key lies in developing personalized approaches that you can maintain consistently while supporting your health, relationships, and career goals. With mindful attention to building sustainable practices, night shift work can become not just manageable but genuinely rewarding over the long term.

Don't miss out!

Visit the website below and you can sign up to receive emails whenever Sarah Chen publishes a new book. There's no charge and no obligation.

https://books2read.com/r/B-A-RFLUC-XXBIF

BOOKS 2 READ

Connecting independent readers to independent writers.

Milton Keynes UK
Ingram Content Group UK Ltd.
UKHW031154251124
451529UK00001B/71

9 798230 016878